COLOURS OF LOVE
in life and after death

COLOURS OF LOVE

in life and after death

Marthie Momberg

PROTEA BOOK HOUSE
PRETORIA
2005

COLOURS OF LOVE
in life and after death

Published in 2000 by Hemel & See Boeke as
"Kleure van liefde – in lewe en sterwe en daarna"
ISBN 0-620-26398-9

First English edition, first impression 2005

Protea Book House
PO Box 35110, Menlopark, 0102
1067 Burnett Street, Hatfield, 0083
protea@intekom.co.za

Typography and design by Tiglix Digital Communication
Cover page by Tiglix Digital Communication
Reproduction by PrePress Images
Printed and bound by Paarl Print

ISBN 1-86919-078-5
© 2005 Marthie Momberg
© All rights reserved. No part of this book may be reproduced
without the permission of the publisher.

Photograph on cover by Hes Range

I dedicate this book to those people who travelled the road with us – our friends, colleagues, family and the medical personnel who assisted us. I do this also on Derik's behalf, as I believe he would have wanted it thus.

Through these people we were able to experience aspects of life that enriched us deeply. But more than anything else, it was the love of each one of these individuals that made us realise that we never needed to fear anything.

I also know that I received Help in my writing – for that, too, my heartfelt thanks.

Marthie Momberg
March 2000

CONTENTS

1. The First Ten Years 9
2. A Clear Day in April 28
3. Now is Always Here 37
4. Pink, White, Green and Deep Purple 52
5. The "Blue" Chemotherapy 75
6. Easter Eggs Filled with Holes 92
7. Antibiotics on an Irrigation Pipe 109
8. "Almost Certainly" 117
9. Completing the First Cycle 134
10. The Turning Point 146
11. A Shift in Time 158
12. The Transition 174
13. Wind, Sun and Finally Mistiness 186
14. The Thoroughfare 194
15. A New Vision 198

Epilogue: The Red Pashmina 208

1

The First Ten Years

I used to find memorial services unbearable. Depressing even. To view the grief of other people, to experience their loss and to accept the finality of death would tear at my very core and leave me nauseous with pain. As I held my own breath on these occasions, I would feel as if life had stopped in me too. I often felt a sense of relief when the ceremony was over.

But this time it was different.

— Original Message —
From: Marthie Momberg
Sent: Saturday, 23 October 1999 21:08 PM
To: Our friends in far places
Subject: Peace

Dear friends
It is Saturday evening. Music from *Jonathan Livingston Seagull* fills the whole house.

When Derik and I started dating in 1977 (we were students at Potch), we often listened to this music together. Derik was gripped by the tale of the seagull – he bought both the cassette and the book, and had seen the film a few times. Then, I did not understand what it was about. It took 22 years before I could listen to the music with the same intensity as he did.

A few weeks ago, a colleague and friend of mine voiced her thoughts to Derik by quoting from *Jonathan Livingston Seagull*. It moved Derik deeply. The incident led me to order the CD for him. The day on which I gave it to him was the last day he was able to listen to music. His hearing had already deteriorated as a result of the abnormal pressure of the blood in his veins. I played the first two tracks for him (and probably for the rest of the neighbourhood as well): "Prologue" and "Be". He was unable to listen to more. The sound waves from the loud music were painful to him.

Yesterday we listened to the music once more. That was when we expressed our thanks for Derik's life. It was one of the most beautiful experiences of my life. I did not want us to mourn in the traditional sense, nor did I want a conventional memorial service, as neither Derik nor I had ever pitied ourselves at any stage. At all times we had felt fulfilled by the process we were going through. That is why the emphasis was on giving thanks.

We combined music with reminiscences and tales by friends, as well as a meditation by Theunis, our minister. As with the thanksgiving Derik and I had had a month before, we lit a round, white candle with three wicks – for faith, love and hope. This time I lit the wicks myself. Theunis's message was that we should all embrace life and enjoy it – just as Derik had done. He also drew on what Derik had said in his thanksgiving message a month before: faith is the historical perspective, since it is about our experience of God; hope is the trust in what God is capable of doing, and is therefore the future perspective; and love provides the present perspective, which is based on the Will of God. Derik had emphasised that it is especially the love of the people who surround us that provides meaning to our lives, because through them we experience the presence of God in a tangible way.

Before the service we played Mozart's Concerto for clarinet and orchestra in A major. This music was used for the soundtrack of *Out of Africa*. It had always reminded Derik of the freedom he experienced while flying. He had often listened to it in the hospital, and also here at home. When Theunis had finished speaking of faith, love and hope, we played the first track from the soundtrack of *Trois Couleurs: Bleu*. This is a musical arrangement of 1 Corinthians 13, composed for the unification of Europe. After the blessing we played "Be" from *Jonathan Livingston Seagull**:

> Lost
> on a painted sky
> where the clouds are hung
> for the poet's eye
> you may find him
> if you may find him
>
> We dance
> to a whispered voice
> overheard by the soul
> undertook by the heart
> and you may know it
> if you may know it
>
> There
> on a distant shore
> by the wings of dreams
> through an open door
> you may know him
> if you may

* Song by Niel Diamond.

While the soul
would become the stone
which begat the spark
turned to living bone
Holy, Holy
Sanctus, Sanctus

Be
as a page that aches for a word
which speaks on a theme
that is timeless
while the sun god will make for your day
sing
as a song in search of a voice
that is silent
and the one God
will make for your way

Then, as now, my heart was overflowing. I thank the Lord for the man with whom I was able to spend more than half of my life thus far. It was a privilege to take leave of him in this way.

I am also grateful that I could be with him at the time of his death. That I could hold him and that we were here in our own home. His death has left a vast emptiness, yet I cannot but admit that I am extremely grateful. There is a peace that transcends all understanding.

EVERLASTING IS THE LOVE OF THE LORD
Psalm 103:15–17

As for man, his days are like grass;
He flourishes like a flower of the field;
for the wind passes over it,

and it is gone,
and its place knows it no more.

> But the steadfast **love** of the **Lord**
> is from **everlasting** to **everlasting**.*

Please share in my peace.
MM

The first time I met Derik there was nothing immediately striking about him. When I brought him home, my parents were, to say the least, unimpressed. According to them, he was not nearly as attractive as my previous boyfriend. He also did not have any notable assets. He was little more than a quiet student with worn "takkies" and a blustery DKW. My parents, who knew that I was very selective about my friends, could not understand what I saw in this man. One of my best friends made it clear that my judgement had failed me. But I ignored them because my soul was at peace from the moment I met Derik.

My friends and family did not remain sceptical for long. My three school-going brothers thought it was great fun to have someone who was willing to rough it with them, build kites, arm wrestle, play chess and later, engage them in earnest conversation. My mother enjoyed being able to provide meals that were enjoyed with great relish, and Derik's practical bent pushed him up a few notches in my father's estimation. They soon discovered that Derik's charm lay in the depth of his being, not in his external appearance.

---

* Unless stated otherwise, all quotations from The Bible taken from the New English Bible, NIV, 1970 edition. Available: http://collections.chadwyck.com.login.ezproxy.library.ualberta.ca/bie/htxview?template=basic.htx&content=frameset.htx

He was – for lack of a better description – my soul mate. Although neither of us was very talkative, we could discuss and analyse issues for hours. When we were quiet, we communicated in other ways. Throughout our relationship and our marriage there was a strong physical attraction. A week or two after we had started dating, I pushed Derik away from me during an embrace and asked him why he had recently been focused only on my physicality! Could we not rather just talk? Eventually we did find a balance.

I did not love him because of his wonderful characteristics – that was only part of the attraction. There are other people who have the same qualities. I knew I belonged with him because his being, his presence, his soul, the sound of his voice, the energy he emitted – call it what you will – had untied my own soul. Contact with him always moved me into a unique "dimension" or experience of feeling. It is difficult to describe my bond with him; I lack sufficient words. It was almost as if I was only truly "at home" with him. My being could relax in his presence; he brought a pervasive sense of peace to me that I did not experience with anyone else. With him I could move closer to myself.

We started dating on 7 June 1977 and got married two-and-a-half years later, on 7 December 1979. We knew from the start that we would always and eventually officially be together. That is why I was rather amused when Derik "asked" me to marry him. It was such a quaint, loveable thing to do. I guess he wanted a formal "yes" before he spent all his savings on an engagement ring.

At the time, he was a student in the Department of Theology at the University of Pretoria, and I was a third-year student at Potchefstroom University. A week after proposing Derik bought a diamond. Then on a Saturday morning, in the sweltering summer heat of Pretoria's city centre, we searched for a suitable setting – almost casually, while running errands.

It was difficult to decide on a ring without a diamond in it. Moreover, my fingers are so thin that we did not have much choice. After choosing the setting, I discovered to my surprise that my friends had spent weeks studying jewellers' catalogues and dreaming of rings before their engagements. Had my choice been too hasty? It did not really bother me. It did not even cross my mind that putting on the ring for the first time is supposed to be a special moment. As far as I was concerned, Derik could have mailed the ring to me in a cardboard box. The bond between us was already in place.

But he always liked to surprise me. A week or so later, in October 1978, he came to Potchefstroom to attend the annual farewell dinner at my residence. He remarked with disappointment that the jeweller had not been able to finish the ring, and that he had hoped to bring it with him. I viewed his disappointment lightly and with a slight smile. The ring was not that important to me. I had been so busy with the final arrangements for the dinner that evening that I had not had time to think about rings. Derik, who loved to liken me to an ant because of my incessant scurrying, was most probably quietly amused at my indifference. He knew that I had no expectations regarding the celebration of our engagement, but he saw to it that we would always remember the occasion.

That evening, just as I had finished my speech (I was the new Head Student) and was sitting down, Derik took my hand and slipped the ring onto my finger during the grace. Of course, I was forced to sit quietly until the formalities had been completed. It was, after all, the 1970s, and we were attending a formal dinner at Potchefstroom University for Christian Higher Education – decorum was highly regarded in those days!

The memory of that evening resurfaced when I received the following e-mail from a university friend in the week following our thanksgiving service for Derik's life:

——Original Message ——
From: TK
Sent: Thursday, 28 October 1999 10:59 PM
To: Marthie Momberg
Subject: RE: Peace

Marthie
Thank you for sharing the precious moments of farewell with us. We are glad that you are experiencing such peace. It is a blessing and we are grateful for it with you.

When people speak of memorable engagements, I have always mentioned your and Derik's engagement. It is something I will always remember: Derik's immense pride at having completed the task. And your total surprise. And then the sparkle in both of your eyes.

Once more, as always… strength.
Regards
Thomas

Our wedding day also came and went without my planning and contemplating the ceremony much. My parents saw to the organisation, partly because I was writing my final examinations in Potchefstroom. My mother eventually had to urge me to choose a dress. In retrospect this seems odd, as I enjoy dressing up and entertaining. All I wanted at the time was to be with Derik.

Derik felt the same and did not bother much about "the other people". To the dismay of many, we spent almost our entire wedding day together doing frivolous things such as watching a James Bond movie. Somewhere someone said something like "On her wedding day, a bride is not supposed to…" but we were already heading through the doorway. An hour or two before the wedding I had a quick bath, got dressed and posed for a short photograph session before the church service.

We had a fairy tale reception in my parents' garden. Three weeks of pouring Transvaal rain had preceded that balmy, windless December evening. The summer garden was beautiful. Giant baskets of flowers were suspended from the trees, and the coloured lights in the branches lit the tables for three hundred guests. My mother had prepared a most delicious meal. It was a wonderful evening with friends and family!

By that time, Derik had, with his father's help, managed to exchange his DKW for a Datsun 1200 van. The idea was that we would travel the roughly fifteen hundred kilometres to Cape Town for our honeymoon in it. On leaving the reception, I was therefore pleasantly surprised when Derik gallantly opened the door of his father's comfortable Mercedes-Benz for me!

One can divide our life together into two broad phases: 1979 to 1989, and 1990 to October 1999. In the first ten years, we got to know ourselves and each other better. This was our *Sturm und Drang* phase in which we studied and moulded each other. The second ten years was a time in which we were able to live out our love for each other without reserve and when we grew to a clearer understanding of who and what we were.

There were many people who found resonance in Derik. During the early years of our marriage this threatened me. I did not know myself then, and his friendships with others heightened my insecurity. I wanted selfishly to claim him for myself. This anxiety, our lack of experience and a mutual stubbornness caused much conflict during that time. The more I tried to rein him in, the more claustrophobic and in need of freedom he felt. It was always important to Derik to live a full life and to try out new things. During the late seventies and eighties, Derik focused on exploring new points of view. He tested and refined his own opinions through his postgraduate studies in theology and psychology, and formed an independent view of life.

The rapid pace and radical way in which he grew in himself threatened me. At that time, I did not question much and I was quite happy with most of society's views. But Derik demanded more from life. He was on an exciting voyage of discovery; I was in rebellion against his change. To me, the fact that our paths no longer ran parallel held the possibility of separation. If I could have, I would have harnessed his thoughts. It was ironic. The more I denied him freedom, the less I was able to "hold" him and it felt as if I was losing him. Because I was struggling at that stage to accept responsibility for my own happiness, I had started living my live through him and had neglected my own talents. Actually, I did not really know what my own ideals and dreams were – they revolved mostly around Derik and our future together. Perhaps that was why it was such a disappointment when we realised that we would never be able to have children together.

My fear that he would die young became an obsession. If he was even slightly late, I would think the worst. It was essential to me always to have him close by, and I could not imagine a life without him – the mere thought filled me with great anguish.

The more I used Derik as a medium through which to experience life, the more I feared life itself. I had indeed reached a point where I was afraid to live. In fact, after the first ten years of our marriage, despite having completed eight degrees and two postgraduate diplomas between the two of us, we – especially I – did not yet know much about life.

Derik encouraged me to realise myself, and not to be dependent on him. He did not want me to love him because I needed him. I gradually came to appreciate his inner strength and discerning abilities. My rebellion against the changes in his thinking diminished, and his views on freedom and happiness began to make sense to me. And yet in the beginning it was not easy to apply these principles to my life.

Towards the end of the 1980s, I decided that my life could not continue like this any longer. I had been teaching and, initially, had been the primary breadwinner while Derik was studying. Later, I continued to teach because I did not believe that I was capable of doing anything else. I had never really enjoyed my work, and had contemplated a career change for years. One day in 1989, in the middle of a class, I decided to draw a line through my teaching career. It was unfair to deny my own desires. I simply had to risk the leap.

My leap was fairly conservative. I wanted to return to the university for a degree that would give me a professional qualification. Without it I did not believe I could make a successful transition. I already held a Master's degree in literature, but now my choice fell on dentistry – to the shock and (justified) amazement of my friends and family. I had never been interested in the natural sciences, had not done physical science in Grade 12 and my knowledge of mathematics was decidedly rusty. Still, I was very excited about being selected for the course, and Derik supported my decision wholeheartedly.

The year 1990 thus rang in the second decade, and a new era, of our lives. We were ready for change and renewal. Perhaps the radical changes in the world also contributed somewhat, since the Berlin Wall fell at that time, and on 2 February 1990, State President FW de Klerk announced that Nelson Mandela would be released from prison. Besides the new doors that were opening within and beyond the borders of our country, the nineties also brought about changes in our immediate environment. The first we became aware of was that Derik's father was diagnosed with an advanced form of cancer. He died a year later, on 2 February 1991.

Initially we were not quite sure where our personal renewal would lead us, but we began by changing our surroundings. My first act after resigning from my teaching position was to change the casually chosen setting of my ring to a more practical, simple design that suited my personal style better. Then I registered as a student in the Faculty of Dentistry at the University of Stellenbosch. Next we decided to replace our house with its long hallway, many bedrooms, two studies, lounge, family and dining rooms for something more suited to two people who could not have children.

By April 1990 we were in the swing of change. Within a single day, shortly before Easter, we sold the house, Derik exchanged his lecturing post at the University of Stellenbosch for a career with a financial institution, and I realised that dentistry was clearly not my direction, and dropped out of the course.

I did not have a job, and was unsure of what I wanted to do, but I had given a few faltering steps in the direction of a new future. I had begun to trust the process of life. Our friends and family also sighed with relief. Since Derik could start in his new position only at the end of the year, we decided to lock up our apartment on the banks of the Eerste River and make use of the study leave the university had granted him. We both accepted scholarships to do postgraduate research in the Netherlands. His field was psychology, mine literature.

However, within weeks Derik had to return to South Africa as a result of his father's illness. He encouraged me to stay abroad, for a while at least. Five months later I was still in the Netherlands without him. It was a safe way of experimenting with freedom. I could do what I wanted, supported by a husband who loved me and longed for me. And so I gradually learned how gratifying it was to be independent. I had also been freed of earthly possessions. My bicycle and my books, my room with its desk, typewriter, bed, two chairs, a coffee table and a vase filled with flowers proved sufficient. I shared kitchen and bathroom facilities with my housemates.

The months alone in Utrecht were cathartic. In the mornings, like many other South African students, I earned extra income by working as a cleaner at the university. While working in one of the natural sciences buildings, I once wrote to a friend about my personal experiences:

3 September 1990

Dear Noëlline

Things are better now.

The mere sight of the Periodic Table against the wall of the Chemistry Department's hallway initially brought my soul to a standstill and would shut my head down. When I also had to clean in the section for Special Dentistry while Miene and Lenie were on leave, my innermost being cried out. I could not contain my audible groans in the consulting rooms and in the section where they store new dentures for people who, for example, had been in accidents. I felt sick to my stomach, almost as if I was experiencing death.

But things are better now.

I am slowly meeting once more the Marthie who likes books and fantasies. I am gradually letting go of the idea of becoming a dentist. I have learned one thing here – that a person can be happy on many different levels. You say you envy me, Noëlline. But the opening up of new worlds also b ings new pain. There is one door I would like to close before I return. My dear husband, who is suffering greatly at the moment, understands this, and has said he can wait until 19 October. I'll be too late for the birth of your child, Derik's birthday, and for spring. But I hope to be in time for a new life. Thank you so much for the peacock feather you sent me. I am well, and hope to hear the same from you.

Lots of love

Marthie

My initial plan had been to return before Derik's birthday in September, but I simply was not ready. I needed more time to close the door on my old life and to make sure that I knew who I was. In the past, I would never have dreamed of being away on Derik's birthday, yet now it seemed acceptable. And, once more, Derik gave me the space to do so. He was excited about the progress I had made within myself and understood why I had delayed my return. For a whole month more, I would be able to think and study, explore the outer reaches of the Netherlands, and spend an entire week hiking through the Forest of the Ardennes.

I started to realise that a person can experience unity and intimacy without one's loved one being physically present. I also began to understand that freedom did not mean a lack of commitment, but that space actually allowed for a greater connection when there was mutual respect and trust between the respective parties. Someone who is free has much more to offer. Derik was no longer my crutch; he was the man I loved, and no more.

Our exchanging of letters during the months apart contributed to our discovering new facets of each other. It often happens that words are the most ineffective means of communication, but in this instance the written word allowed us to say things to each other in a very direct manner. Our telephone conversations were not nearly as fulfilling as our letters. Unlike speech, a letter can be read again and again. One can put it on the table while drinking tea and rest one's hand on the envelope; one can place it under the pillow while sleeping. We knew we loved each other before our short separation. Now we began to see why.

From that time on, we consciously chose to be with each other every day. We never again took our relationship nor our marriage for granted simply because we had said some vows ten years earlier. We began to encourage each other as separate individuals, had fewer fears, and thus grew closer together. We realised that we were not married to replicas of each other, but that two individuals could form a team that could achieve far more as a unit than individually. It was precisely the other person's perspective that contributed to a more rounded, greater experience. We were together out of choice and for sheer pleasure, and not because we needed to lean on each other, had to nurse each other or maintain some or other commitment.

Returning to my husband in South Africa was exciting. Although we lived in the Cape at the time, he and a friend surprised me on my arrival at the airport in Johannesburg before I had to board my connecting flight. I remember how the three of us drove to his parents' home and how I did not register a single word of the conversation. I just kept looking at him. In the preceding months we had written to each other very intimately; now we were together in real flesh. It was something completely different. I could not stop looking at him. After a brief visit to my in-laws, we left for a hotel where we spent the night.

It was almost like the time when we had lived on the then "Border". Ruacana was a tiny town on the dusty plateau of Sector 10, Ovamboland, where Derik was to be stationed as a service chaplain during the Namibian War in the early eighties. We had chosen to go and live in this outpost for two years. It was a way of saving money while exploring new territory. We both enjoyed taking risks, and we wanted to venture into the "unknown". I had been fortunate to get a teaching post at the local primary school, and because I had had to start teaching, I had to spend the first six weeks alone in Ruacana while Derik completed his officers' course in Pretoria. I waited for Derik in the house with its bomb shelter, orange lounge furniture, broken stove, barber spiders, gauze windows and garden with ten paw-paw trees.

But Derik knew how to get things done. He let me know that he would come to visit for a weekend. One of my colleagues at the school subtly tried to warn me that I should not count on this happening. She explained that the military aeroplanes from Waterkloof to Ondangwa were always very full and that it was almost impossible to find space on them. One needed authorisation from those in high command since these planes were used for military purposes, not weekend jaunts. The Rum Run (the supply plane transporting soldiers from Ondangwa to Ruacana three times a week) was seldom on time, she said, which meant that what did not get done by Friday had to wait until Monday. She pointed out that there would not necessarily be transport from the airfield into town, even if the Rum Run did manage to land. In fact, it would be better if I did not bank on seeing Derik that weekend. But I continued to count the days on my calendar. I believed that he would arrive; Derik was someone I could count on.

And he did arrive – at our borrowed home on that Friday afternoon, in a cloud of white dust on the back of an army truck, wearing his "browns". And just as I did not hear the conversation on the road from the airport eight years ago, unable to keep my eyes off Derik, so again I could not tear my eyes away from him that afternoon in Ruacana. He sat on the orange sofa, in brown boots with innumerable buckles, feet together and knees wide apart. We talked, but all I could think of was how I was going to untie those dusty buckles and buttons fast enough.

Years later, after my return from Utrecht in October 1990, we sat like that again in the chairs of the hotel room and talked. Neither of us heard a thing then; both of us were merely looking. It was part of our foreplay. We deliberately spun out and savoured the first taste of each other. This is how he had described his feelings to me while I was still in the Netherlands:

17 September 1990
Stellenbosch

Hallo my love
Tonight I am filled with a sense of ambivalence. On the one hand, I do not mind your being away. But on the other hand, I truly wish you were here. I miss your bodily presence and warmth. Take note: yours, and not any other woman's. I surely have more than enough time now to take a good look at the other side of the fence, but that is not what I desire. I long for your body, your conversation, your humour – your totally-different-to-me being. I yearn for your closeness and being-there, even your silences beside me that contain a specific, non-verbal communication. The understanding in your eyes, the support/sounding board for my schemes/theories.

> At night I search for you beside me in bed.
> I want to slide my hand over your soft warm body…
> Want to stroke your breasts into erect peaks
> that strain upwards, strain out, purely boisterous,
> to where pain-pricks mingle with the pleasure of surrender.
>
> Let my hand slip across your rib-taken-from-man,
> hips, pubis.
> My fingers tangle in your bush, portal
> to experienced human bliss.
> Veins, stretched wide, distended
> unrushed at own pace reveal
> the desire to strain, to urge,
> to bring climax in transito.

Open-inviting-warm-smooth
the member in hidden captivity enclosed
with
shallow breaths
white-fingered knuckle-fists
head-thrown-back-straining
open-mouthed gasp for breath
receive with surging the power-pleasure
of being together, in one another
forced without choice to rubicon.

In the afterglow of the resurrection
the swell withered to nothingness
the valley to closure
experience perfection.

In hazy ecstasy
sweat-ridden bodies
we slumber,
hands knitted together, legs entwined
with satisfaction and completion
postlude circling into prelude
for the next symphony...

Yes, if only you were here, that which is on paper could be played out/lived. Would it not be heavenly-joyful for you too?

Sorry for not writing a nice chatty letter, or a compilation of my day-to-day activities. At this point, my reason is governed completely by my emotions and desires. I will write again later in the week, a letter that will be more easily digestible/manageable than this one.
Me-and-me

About a month later, on the evening of 18 October 1990, I left Holland to arrive in South Africa the next day, 19 October 1990.

In the first months after my return, we could not get enough of each other. During the week Derik worked in Cape Town and I did freelance editing, but on the weekends we went to secluded places along the West Coast and the Cape South Coast, where we enjoyed each other, and laughed and played. We bought a plot in Paradyskloof, Stellenbosch, and began to plan our new house that had to surround us with light and warmth, yet also have enough space for friends and large, wide verandas for relaxing. It was as if we were building a new life together. The nineties, we knew, would be filled with good things for us. We looked forward to the change and new direction. But we did not know then that besides Derik's father, also my father, Derik's sister and many of our friends and family would pass on during this time. Derik, too, took leave of this life during the night of 18 October 1999 and entered a new life early in the morning of 19 October 1999. It was exactly nine years after my return from Utrecht.

2

A Clear Day in April

It was my mother who for months had remarked that she was worried about Derik. She sensed that there was something amiss with him. I myself became increasingly restless towards the end of 1997 and was plagued by acute and continuous inner feelings of unease. It felt as if I was not paying attention to the right things, and I was also unusually tired and burdened. Despite the fact that just about everything was going well for me – I had a fulfilling job, a happy marriage, good friends and enough money – I was searching for a deeper sense of satisfaction and I had no idea how to achieve this. It was as if I had outgrown myself, but lacked the ability to burst out of my casing. I was not sure where I was heading, but knew my search was related to a desire for more freedom, a broader perception – a more intense experience of life itself.

At night I dreamed repeatedly about water. There were giant waves that threatened me and people I knew (mostly Derik and our immediate family). Typical of these dreams was that none of these waves ever engulfed us. Before this could happen, I would either wake up or the dream would end. I therefore did not know what the outcome of the dreams was going to be. At times I was vaguely aware that the water would not submerge us, but I did not know what would prevent this from happening. Once I dreamt that I had to lead a large crowd of people, including one of my brothers, away from this watery hazard. We had to follow an extremely long and tedious detour through the interior, but eventually we reached safety.

At the time, Derik and I were working hard, too hard, and we were both forty-something. We felt weary and discontented, but thought that this was typical of our circumstances. Anyway, it is quite acceptable in our society for people to work hard at this age. We blamed our careers and started to hate the tempo at which we worked. Both of us regularly commuted to other cities for business, and thus we were seldom home together during the week. Over the weekends, we were so exhausted that we started to avoid visiting friends. We also neglected our families. It felt as if we never had time to climb mountains, discover new places, to read or to laugh. We didn't feel good about ourselves, and this lifestyle no longer made any sense to us. We were giving too much and not investing enough in ourselves. We were merely doing, and no longer experiencing.

Like so many people, we compromised and fitted in with what we thought life expected from us. We were becoming like those who constantly complain about having too much work and too little time, yet nonetheless toil on day after day, grateful to collapse into bed at night. However, this was not the whole truth. What we did not know was that we were so utterly tired because there was something physically wrong with us.

Late one Wednesday evening I erupted. It was supposed to have been the first night in a long time that we would be together during the week. We had been looking forward to it. Derik had to attend a short function after work, and would be home in time for dinner. But it was after eleven when he finally got home. He was excited, as he had, during the course of the evening, recruited two people to help him at work. This would bring relief, as he could no longer cope with his workload.

I was furious because he was so late, but more than anything else, I felt that we were heading for an unavoidable disaster. Yet again we had tried to arrange an evening together, and yet again our work had spoiled our plans. It felt as if our lives had spun out of control, and that is exactly how I behaved that evening. I did not even give him an opportunity to explain; I simply ranted on. I tried to convey my immeasurable frustration with livid gesticulations, raging words and tears. In the end, he also cried with me – and told me that he was so tired he wished he could die.

We realised we had to change our circumstances. That was inevitable. We were not satisfied with a life that was being determined by the demands of society. We had seen too often how people's lives had been cut short too soon. Two of our friends and a cousin had recently passed away, and Derik's sister had also died shortly before. We knew that we wanted to enjoy every moment of our lives together, we wanted to laugh and play together again. We also knew that this would not happen by itself, but that we would have to make choices. We had no one but ourselves to blame for our current circumstances. If we had been working too hard or not been paying attention to the right things, it was because we had allowed it to become like this. Frankly, it was time to take control of our lives again.

Just as we had had to reconsider our priorities at the end of the eighties, we now had to take stock again, make changes to our lifestyle and set new goals. Previously, our immaturity had stood in the way of a perfect relationship. Now we had arrived at this perfection in our relationship, but neither of us had the energy to enjoy it to the full. That evening, as we sat on the stairs in our house, we formulated our plan of action. This plan would require incisive adjustments from both of us, including career changes. The first step was to take a holiday and to rest thoroughly.

Since both of us were sick of travelling, we decided to spend our holiday at home and regain our strength. We wanted to breathe deeply once more, go for walks in the mountains and vineyards surrounding our house, have coffee in town, visit friends, and enjoy the tranquil beauty of Stellenbosch. We would consciously not do anything, but simply experience and get in touch with ourselves again.

The break also gave Derik an opportunity to visit a doctor. He had already been perspiring abnormally for more than a month, and Rieksie, our aromatherapist, had mentioned to him that his spleen was enlarged.

It was the first weekend in April 1998. I remember that clear autumn morning vividly. It was the first day of our holiday. After his appointment with the doctor, Derik went to the hospital for blood tests. Later, in the town centre, we slowly strolled in the dappled shade of the oak trees along Andringa Street, past all our favourite Saturday morning spots: The Dorp Street Gallery, the quaint shops, then left into Church Street to our favourite Dutch coffee shop. Along the way, we passed a dear friend, Henk, with his sun-bleached blonde hair. Our hands briefly touched in passing as we smiled and greeted each other. I was wearing my blue blouse and my wide khaki pants. My arm was hooked in Derik's.

Over a cup of coffee, Derik casually told me what the doctor had said. His symptoms could indicate a number of conditions – anything from an infection or malaria to liver disease or cancer. Our conversation in the coffee shop, and later that afternoon as we drove along the beautiful mountainous coastline on the winding road to our friends in Hangklip, was filled with silences, yet it was intense. We spoke of our dreams for times to come. We were desperate for a radical change. Both of us wanted to help other people to heal, emotionally and physically. We also wanted to write – Derik in particular had felt strongly about this for a while. A few weeks earlier, I had concluded that it would be best to resign from my job and was therefore at the time training to become an estate agent in an attempt to have more free time. Today I know that that career change seemed to offer me a solution then, but it had never been a dream. Just as I had started the course in dentistry nine years before only to discover that it was not really my direction, I was again about to qualify myself for a new career, this time to discover that one cannot find satisfaction in something if one's heart is not in it. We therefore spoke about our dreams: about our future together. The possibility of a serious illness was not a reality.

That evening at dinner Derik was quiet and did not eat much. We went to bed early. Just before we switched off the light, I asked Derik to repeat what the doctor had said to him. We held each other and slept.

Early the next morning we returned home as other friends were waiting there for us. On our arrival they relayed a message from the doctor: we had to call him urgently. We knew that it was serious. We returned his call, and he was at our house within ten minutes.

Derik and I sat on the veranda with him. Looking straight at us, the doctor told us that Derik's white blood count was abnormally high and that he definitely had leukaemia. He could not tell which kind yet, but he had already booked a bed in the hospital for Derik so that further tests could be done. We had to leave immediately as the specialist was already waiting for us. We walked Johann, the doctor, to his car to say goodbye. The sky was a clear blue. My husband comforted me.

From Derik's diary:
(My dearest wife, I have decided to keep a diary of my experiences, feelings and thoughts while I have the time. Hopefully we will be able to read it together one day and enjoy life fully once more.)

March 1998
Just after eight on the morning of 11 March, Chris called me at work to tell me that Alta had passed away. As I was driving home, the grey rain curtain of the Western Cape cried with me over yet another heart-rending reality of life. We are born only to die again.

For the rest of March, I sweated even more at night, and I felt exhausted. I recall how I sat on the steps and told you that I felt so tired that I wished I'd die. Was it a prophecy or self-fulfilment?

April 1998
"Man, actually I have bad news for you. The blood tests have confirmed that you have leukaemia."

For a moment I felt as if I was hearing these words from outside my own body. My wife, our doctor friend and I were sitting on the veranda when Johann said these words. It was 5 April 1998, one week before Easter Sunday. How ironic. We were celebrating Christ's resurrection from the dead, and I had received my death sentence. Or at least, that's what I thought.

It was a lovely day in Stellenbosch. Our bodies baked in the warm sun, and one was aware of the perfection of God's creation. The roses spread the full glory of their colour and fragrance in the sunlight. On the bench, our black cat, Katerina, stretched herself with great delight on the quilt. It was an almost perfect day.

"What does this mean to us?" my wife asked. Only then did I become aware of the anything but perfect announcement. Leukaemia. What did it mean? I knew it meant cancer of the blood, but I lacked any further knowledge. Our doctor started explaining carefully, but quickly added that leukaemia was not his field of specialisation, and that such cases were usually referred to a haematologist. He had already made an appointment with the specialist, and if I agreed, I would be hospitalised that same day. On Monday they would do a bone marrow biopsy in order to make a final diagnosis.

When the doctor had left, my wife and I remained standing in our driveway. Slowly I became aware of her sobs. I wanted to comfort her, but I did not know how. What should I say? What was I to do? What effect was this disease going to have on our lives? And I was not even feeling sick yet! I had only gone to the doctor because I was feeling so extremely tired. I still believed that I was only exhausted from working too hard. I ascribed the nightly sweats to the fact that we had buried my sister two weeks before. She had also suffered from cancer, like my father who had died a few years before. Was it hereditary?

The rest of Sunday was a blur.

After the doctor had left, we returned to the veranda in a dumbfounded daze. Our friends brought us warm, sweet tea. We conveyed the message to them haltingly, packed a few belongings and left for the hospital in Bellville. By Monday evening, after a painful bone marrow biopsy, we knew that Derik was suffering from chronic myeloid leukaemia (CML). According to the specialist, he had been ill for at least six to eight months, as his leukocyte count was extremely high.

It is the rarest of the four types of leukaemia. Normally, a person's bone marrow (a sponge-like tissue in the major bones of the body) produces three kinds of blood cells: white blood cells that attend to the immune system; red blood cells that convey oxygen; and blood platelets that help with clotting. In the case of CML, the bone marrow produces too many white blood cells, which often invade other organs like the liver or the spleen, causing the organ to swell and malfunction. On the other hand, the white blood cells no longer reach maturity, which means that they cannot function properly.

People who suffer from CML also clearly have an abnormal chromosome in one, or all, of the leukaemia cells. It is called the Philadelphia chromosome and is distinguished by the fact that the ninth and the twenty-second chromosomes exchange places, thus forming an abnormal gene. This abnormality develops as part of the disease and is apparently not hereditary.

People who are exposed to high levels of radiation, like the survivors of the nuclear bombs in Japan, or people who have been exposed to X-rays too often have a slightly greater tendency to develop the disease. There are also suggestions that other factors, such as exposure to chemicals and viruses, can lead to CML, but as yet there is no proof of this.

According to the doctor, the chronic phase of the disease could last between three and four years. This would typically be followed by a year-long blast phase and an acute phase, which would last a few weeks. According to the haematologist, the expected three to four years, or perhaps even ten years if Derik responded well to treatment, left us with more than enough time before the disease would take it's toll. We were to be thankful that he did not have acute myeloid leukaemia (AML), as that would have given him no more than a few weeks to live.

But what are three, four or even ten years when one is planning a lifetime together? If one felt that one was on the verge of an exciting, new phase of life? This was not what we had expected to hear. It was extremely difficult to share this news with the rest of the family so soon after the death of Alta, whom we had all loved dearly.

Derik wanted confirmation of the facts before he told his family, and he also wanted to wait until he was home before contacting them. It was only on the afternoon before his discharge that I drove to my own mother to tell her. Little did I know that she had already received the news via the grapevine. She held me tightly while I cried out, my body jerking from shock, and eventually I was able to tell her that my husband was very, very ill.

After three days in hospital, Derik returned home with bags full of pills and the hope of living for a few years.

To me, autumn has always been the most beautiful time of the year in the Boland. It was the perfect season in which to try to come to terms with the news – the bright, quiet air during the day, a chill on one's back in the evening and the mistiness of the early morning accompanied by the plovers' hoarse cries. One by one we told our friends. They held us and cried with us. We were not rebellious; rather, we felt rudderless.

We were together at home for a portion of that April, as we had planned. We went for walks in the mountains and vineyards around our home, took deep breaths, had coffee in town, visited with friends, and took in the beauty of Stellenbosch. Pieter, one of my brothers, came down from Pretoria to be with us for the Easter weekend.

On Easter Monday, my brother Louis and his family joined the rest of us for lunch. I had bought enormous Easter eggs for the children, which we hid in the garden. In the end, no one had a chance to eat the chocolates, for Derik used his own "magic" to make the eggs appear and disappear, over and over again.

A sense of unreality characterised that afternoon that was filled with delightful laughter as we watched Derik's tricks in amazement. We experienced his games and the clear autumn day as if through a haze, from a distance. Our actual experiences were not visible. We first had to give form to our true thoughts and feelings on a deep personal level before we could allow them to surface.

3

Now is Always Here

Derik's illness affected his daily life enormously. He had to stop running; he could no longer go deep sea diving; he had to stop his flying lessons, he was not even allowed to mow the lawn. His white blood count was so high (156 instead of somewhere between 4 and 11) that he could suffer a thrombosis attack if he did any exercise. No regular exercise meant that Derik had to make radical adaptations to his lifestyle.

Ever since I had known him, and even before, Derik had participated in sport. He was a long-distance runner, went diving, played underwater hockey, sailed, glided, practised karate, and played rugby and squash. Not being allowed to fly affected him most of all. He was on the verge of getting his licence, and already co-owned an aeroplane with four other people. But he faced up to his reality squarely. That it was a great loss to him is unquestionable. Yet he never brooded over it, and never complained. To him this situation was merely an unpleasant fact. No more.

We wrestled with other questions. Rational and irrational thoughts criss-crossed our minds. How had it happened that Derik had contracted leukaemia? According to the doctor it was not hereditary, but what did it indicate when the third person from the same family contracted cancer within eight years? What had caused his system to deteriorate? Could it have been the fast foods that had replaced our normal diet during our recent trip to North America? I had missed our regular quota of fresh fruit and vegetables enormously – could this have affected Derik as well? How rundown had his system become after running the Comrades? Was it the stress of his work that had finally taken its toll? Why had he never felt really well again after he had had an abscess in his tooth treated? How could we be sure that the low-level X-rays at airport departure lounges had not had an effect on him? Why did we know so many people in Stellenbosch and Somerset West who had cancer, or more specifically, blood and lymph node infections? How much poison were we inhaling daily when we walked through the vineyards adjoining our neighbourhood? Had the chemical fire that had raged a few kilometres from our home at the end of 1992 perhaps had a long-term effect? Why, oh why, had he become ill? Why now when we wanted to arrange our lives to suit us better? So sick that his DNA structure had been altered?

During this time we read many books in our search for an explanation of the illness. Numerous writers stated that there are visible correlations between thoughts, emotions and the well-being of the human body. We had personally never doubted that a person's thoughts and predisposition could influence his or her concrete reality. (Our thoughts are, after all, energy, and if there is enough energy of a particular kind, it forms matter.) Yet some writers also pointed out that in a small percentage of people, illness could not be explained by such theories.

Derik was brutally honest with himself and did a thorough self-analysis in his attempt to explain and understand his condition. He did identify, acknowledge and address a single problem in his life, but it was not as if this issue was extraordinarily large. However, it was something that affected him deeply. Yet if I compare his problem to some of the crises experienced by other people, his was not significantly bigger, more profound, or more hidden. Furthermore, he had only this one issue to address, and not a myriad of issues like the rest of us, including me. Over the years, many people have remarked that Derik was the most integrated person they have ever known. Our families, our friends and I have agreed on this. I could not help thinking that, to my knowledge, he was the one person on earth who had the least unfinished business. Despite this, he became very, very ill. Why?

If it is true that we are on earth to learn some or other lesson, one could argue that the sick person is being "punished", or, at least, has to "learn" the hard way. Well-intentioned remarks by some people implied that someone like Derik who had a dreaded disease such as cancer had a greater lesson to learn than those of us who merrily wander about the earth in good health. But if we are to accept that a serious illness always indicates a significant gap in the emotional or spiritual dimension of the sick person, are we not being judgemental? Are we not awakening unnecessary feelings of guilt?

According to the systemic theory that was so close to Derik's heart, and on which he built his clinical therapy and later also his business principles, there is always interplay between the individual and his environment. That is why we are not isolated from those around us; we all affect one another. We cannot point a finger at others without including ourselves: we are a part of the disease, part of the process, part of the reaction to it.

The question is to what extent do we influence each other and our own selves? Are we solely responsible for shaping our own reality and that of those around us? Can I simply wish to become the president of the country and expect my wish to come true within ten years? What if there are a hundred people in the country with the same idea? Do we bring illness, poverty, exploitation, oppression, loss and pain upon ourselves? To my knowledge, no one wittingly asks for these things to befall him or her. On the contrary, we all have other, definite dreams that include positive experiences like happiness, fulfilment, health and prosperity.

If we then do not desire negative things for ourselves, and yet believe that we exert an influence over our reality, does it mean that the desire for these so-called negative experiences, such as sickness and poverty, are located so deep within us that we are not even aware of them? For despite our positive wishes for ourselves, misfortune does still occur.

If we do indeed harbour hidden negative desires within us, it could mean that we have been delivered into a predestined life over which we have no influence. If we follow this logic, then it does not matter what we wish for ourselves, what is destined to happen will happen. At this point I feel that the whole argument becomes somewhat ridiculous, since on the one hand mankind determines his own reality in all respects, yet on the other is unaware of what is being determined (somewhat like a pre-programmed machine), and the outcome may not necessarily agree with his conscious choice. Thus one ends up where one would rather not be, which means that we are passive travellers through life!

Derik and I argued in circles: it was obvious that man does not determine his own reality completely. Conversely, we remained unconvinced that we are delivered to a destiny without a will, that we are mere victims who observe what happens to us and those around us. In any event, where does God fit into such a picture? Who actually creates this reality? Man? Circumstance? God? A combination of all of the above? And who is responsible for what? It was not easy to come to a meaningful conclusion regarding the cause of the disease. There were too many questions. Derik was unable to accept that it was his own (even unconscious) desire to develop leukaemia. He investigated and considered different theories, but in the end decided that he had a physical illness that needed to be treated on a physical level. He also decided to deliberately engage his spiritual and emotional energy to create favourable circumstances for his physical healing.

Personally, I continued to believe the positive aspects of the argument for a while, namely that we create our own reality and that nothing is therefore impossible. And that is why I believed that Derik would be healed completely. I did not yet understand that there is a difference between creating one's own reality and influencing one's own reality. I would only reach this insight in time.

At this stage, a few weeks after his diagnosis, we accepted that we could not explain why Derik had become ill. What we did know was that it was important to distinguish between the cause, or causes, that led to leukaemia, and our managing the effect it would have on our lives. That Derik was ill was a fact. There was no sense in trying to find someone or something to blame. Instead of looking back, we had to look forward. We had to decide what to do with this reality.

Victor Frankl's story of his survival in a German concentration camp strengthened our view that one can choose how to react to a particular situation. Frankl's will-power, deliberate choices and determination had had a profound effect on both of us when we had read his book shortly after our marriage. We had had almost twenty years in which to "practise" not being victims and to accept responsibility for our spiritual well-being. Now we were faced with the biggest challenge of our lives to date.

We therefore consciously decided, firstly, to look for the positive in this situation; secondly, never to pity ourselves, and, thirdly, not to become engulfed by whatever happened. But it was not easy. We realised in the following months that we were sometimes able to achieve these goals, and that at other times we would virtually fall apart.

At the end of April we both returned to work as our holiday was over. It was now time for focused action.

We started finding out as much as possible about Derik's illness. Since the specialist did not have any information on hand that we would be able to "understand", we read anything we could lay our hands on. In our free time we surfed the Internet. At night, we crawled into bed with piles of printouts on chronic and acute myeloid leukaemia, since CML would develop into an acute disease in a few years' time. Night after night we read, and occasionally shared facts. But mostly we sat beside each other in silence, buried in our separate piles of paper. Then we would switch off the lights, say goodnight and sleep. Each of us kept hoping that by chance we alone had read the disturbing facts, and that the other held the good news in his or her hands.

Gradually the picture unfolded: CML represents approximately twenty per cent of all the different types of leukaemia. We read about the symptoms and treatment of the chronic, the blast and the acute phases of this leukaemia. The first task was to bring the high leukocyte count that is usually diagnosed at the start of CML under control. Derik was already being treated for this and was responding well to the treatment.

According to the literature, chemotherapy and the use of alpha-interferon can retard the illness, but cannot cure it. At this stage, CML could only be cured by a bone marrow transplant.

There are three kinds of transplants: the first involves the patient's own bone marrow; the second uses the bone marrow of a sibling with exactly the same genetic composition, and the third relies on the bone marrow of an unrelated donor who has a corresponding genetic structure. If the patient's own bone marrow cannot be used, it is preferable to look at using that of a bother or sister rather than that of an unrelated donor because of the high risks involved in the procedure. Without a transplant, the patient seldom survives for more than the expected three to four years of the chronic phase. A small group of patients react negatively to the medication and do not even live that long.

In the case of a CML patient who does not have a transplant, the chronic phase is followed by a blast phase and then a short acute phase, after which the patient dies. The cause of death is often something like renal failure, excessive bleeding or thrombosis.

This was a disturbing message. The haematologist who was treating Derik explained that the technique of using the patient's own bone marrow was still too new and dangerous. The risk involved in a transplant from a non-related donor was also too big to make it worth considering this option. He finally added that finding a suitable unrelated donor would be highly unlikely. It is more difficult to find corresponding bone marrow than it is to find a replacement heart, lung or kidney that will be accepted by the host's body, since the DNA structure has to match. In any event, according to him, South Africa no longer had a bone marrow bank.

Derik had only one surviving sibling and consequently his chance of finding a related donor was slim. The specialist arranged to have his sister's blood sent from Pretoria to Cape Town so that they could, through a series of complicated tests, determine whether her bone marrow would be suitable. The initial tests indicated that her bone marrow type did not correspond with Derik's. This was obviously a huge disappointment.

As far as we could establish, the haematologist was highly recommended, and according to him, there was yet an alternative treatment. He had been treating patients with high doses of alpha-interferon, with a fair amount of success. Some of his patients had already survived for ten years with a good quality of life. The doctor reckoned that Derik had a forty percent chance of recovery with this medication.

The good news was that Derik's leukocyte count improved from week to week. Every Monday morning before work he went to have his blood tested and every Monday afternoon we received the results. April, May and June passed with Derik making good progress. By the beginning of July, his count was normal and he felt relatively strong and energetic. At this point, we had no reason to question the specialist's recommendation and accepted that Derik would start using alpha-interferon in August.

However, the doctor first wanted to take a two-week break. This also gave us a chance to come to our senses – our April break had not been much of a holiday. We had had a few difficult months and felt the need for rest and peace. Some friends offered to let us use their house on their parents' farm in the Little Karoo, and we accepted their offer with gratitude. We wanted to spend a week there, and an additional few days at a nearby guest-house.

Both of us were looking forward to getting away from doctors' waiting rooms and hospitals and to having only open countryside around us. We planned to leave on the Sunday afternoon. On the Friday after work, I bought a huge pile of fresh fruit and vegetables, and also an assortment of spoils for our Karoo holiday. We wanted to isolate ourselves, but had no intention of lacking anything. That evening a friend prepared a lovely dinner of salads, vegetable dishes and couscous at our house. We drew three chairs around the fireplace and enjoyed an evening of pleasant conversation and good food. It was just the right thing at the start of our holiday.

As we were getting ready for bed later, Derik asked me in passing whether we should not perhaps rather go to Mombasa for our holiday. Mombasa? Why there, I asked. He reminded me that he had gone to buy milk earlier in the evening and that he had, by chance, seen an advertisement in the window of a new travel agency. There was a special offer on a week's stay in Mombasa. A few years previously we had enquired into a trip to Kenya and Tanzania, but eventually had not gone there. So why not go now? Yes, I replied, why not go now? We switched off our bedside lights, cuddled up to each other and fell asleep.

The following morning we woke up just as peacefully. Later, when we could think clearly, we remembered our plans to go to Mombasa. We had not planned or budgeted for a holiday of this nature, but we cast caution to the wind. There was no harm in finding out more about the tour package. But first, a quick trip to the hospital to have Derik's blood tested – just so that we knew exactly what was happening. And in any event, even if we went to the Karoo, we would not be able to get to the pathologist on Monday. And so it happened that we walked into the travel office near our house at eleven o'clock that Saturday morning.

We explained to the owner that we were interested in the offer of a trip to Mombasa. Let's talk, he said in a most welcoming tone. He pointed out that there were also other special offers, particularly to the Orient. Would we perhaps be interested in those instead? Unfortunately, the agent who specialised in foreign travel was not in the office, but if we would come by on Monday morning, she would be there – would that suit us? When did we intend to leave?

Of course, we wanted to leave immediately. Both of us had only two weeks' leave, and, technically, we were already on holiday. There was no time to lose. The friendly agent therefore referred us to the company's branch in a neighbouring town. We would have to hurry, since it was already past eleven, and the agency closed at one. In our haste, we forgot to collect Derik's test results, and halfway to Somerset West we had to turn back to fetch them. The counts were perfect. They could not have been better. We were hastily en route to an exotic holiday. Anyway, who would want to stay here and freeze in the Little Karoo in the middle of July?

It was already half past twelve when we walked into the travel agency, straight into the very efficient hands of Melanie. She wanted to know where we wanted to go. The Maldives? Bali? When she heard that we wanted to leave immediately, and that we could not wait for visas, we decided on Thailand. (Where exactly was Thailand? And what does one do there?) By now, it was already after one o'clock. The agency's door was closed, and all the other staff members had left. Melanie calmly sat with us, analysed our needs and then inserted a CD into her computer. She told us where we should go, what it looked like and what we could do there. We agreed wholeheartedly. It sounded very exciting.

However, the reservations would have to wait until Monday. Melanie had to fly to a conference in Johannesburg on Monday, but promised that she would make the reservations (travel plan, tickets, hotel bookings, etc.) from the Johannesburg branch early on Monday morning. We thanked her once again. It all sounded quite wonderful. We at least knew that Bangkok was the capital of Thailand, but we had never heard of Chiang Mai, Phuket and Samui. But it did not matter, for she seemed to know exactly what we felt like doing.

And so it was. Forty-eight hours later, at lunchtime on Monday, she called us with the final costs and the accommodation arrangements. We were sitting on our bed, surrounded by pamphlets covered in pictures of white beaches and turquoise seas. Melanie's call had made the fantasy a sudden reality.

With the travel plans, expenses and all other arrangements finalised by telephone, we immediately left for town to sort out our finances, buy a hat for Derik, and, of course, tanning lotion.

Early on Tuesday morning, our good friend Piet Grobler dropped us off at the airport. He took a photo of us outside the departures terminal with our arms around each other –

there we stood, extremely excited with two small suitcases, my wide-brimmed straw hat and a brown leather daypack.

I am not sure whether we simply wanted to convince ourselves, or whether it was a spontaneous thought, but we kept assuring each other that this was a good idea. We had the time and the energy to do it now, and after all, we had no idea what lay ahead for us. So we therefore justified exceeding our budget for a trip to Thailand. In the coming months it became clear that it was truly the best thing we could have done for ourselves at the time.

It was one of the happiest holidays of our lives, and certainly the best overseas holiday we ever had. On all our previous travels, we had gone for as long as and as far as our finances would allow (which usually was not very far!). But now we could simply relax for two weeks and enjoy ourselves while other people waited on us. We woke up just before six every morning, and by half past six we had already gone for a walk or a swim. It was a very special time of the day, since we were generally alone on the beach at that hour. After our walk, we would have breakfast and go on some or other interesting day trip with our personal guide. It was an idyllic holiday filled with snorkelling, canoeing, temple visits, elephant rides, shows, reflecting on a different culture and savouring delicious food.

Derik was fit and strong, and our deep care for each other was apparently quite visible. The staff at the hotel on the island of Phuket must have contacted their sister hotel in Samui, for when we arrived on the last island of our visit, we were welcomed to our room with a brightly coloured, overly decorated cake, with the words "Happy Honeymoon" neatly inscribed on it in screaming pink and shocking green. Beside it stood an equally over-dressed statue of a western bride and groom. We fell about laughing and took a photo of the cake and the statue.

Time stood still once more. The two-week experience would become an inexhaustible source of memory to us.

Almost a year later, two days before Derik was finally discharged from the hospital because, according to the doctor, there was nothing more anyone could do for him, the memory of one of our experiences in Thailand carried him through his intense pain. The previous night he had been given a dose of morphine because every cell in his body ached. In particular, his lungs ached terribly when he coughed. During yet another coughing fit, I could no longer stand by and watch his suffer. Silently, I called for help from within my body and from without, and also from Above: "Please HELP him!" Almost immediately Derik's face lit up and he smiled broadly while still clutching his chest. His pain did not diminish, but in that instant he thought of our most memorable meal in the north of Thailand. He said: "Do you remember that great meal we had in…?" There was no need to complete the sentence. I knew exactly what he was referring to.

It had been in Chiang Mai, the city known as "The Rose of the North". We were on our way to the night bazaar and were planning to have dinner at the same restaurant as the night before. It was situated in a clean shopping centre, and the food looked "safe", which is to say, fairly recognisable. (We had to be careful about what we ate, because under no circumstances could Derik risk feeling unwell.)

As we were walking along, someone stuffed a pamphlet into our hands. I did not even look at it, as I was too interested in everything around me. However, a few blocks further, Derik tugged at my sleeve and asked whether we should try the restaurant that was advertised on the small piece of blue and white paper. He pointed to the words that were printed on the back of the pamphlet for the Whole Earth Restaurant. It was these words, in the typically broken English of the Thais, that made us turn around:

EATING FOR ENLIGHTENMENT

Every fiber of food we eat has within it the total
potentiality of cosmic intelligence.
"No matter what we eat, a stressed physiology will not
make the best of it. But eating when free from stress,
create a more valuable chemistry that produces better
perception, which allows for a greater evaluation
of the objects of perception that makes
those objects more charming, appreciation grows,
producing more love, which
in turn cultures the heart." *Maharishi*

Let us be together
Let us eat together
Let us be vital & radiate truth together
We shall not denounce anyone
Never entertain negativity.

88 Sridonchai Road, A. Muang, Chiang Mai

We knew who Maharishi was, and the message made sense to us: there is a connection and an interaction between a positive disposition, the preparation of a meal, the eating and experiencing of it, the thoughts that flow from it and – once more – the disposition. We therefore turned immediately and walked back up the few dusty blocks to where (coincidentally?) I had already noticed the turn-off to the restaurant the previous day. And we were not disappointed!

Maharishi Maheshi Yogi is the person who introduced the technique of Transcendental Meditation (TM) to the western world. It is a specific type of meditation that is not linked to a particular religion. It involves a mental technique that enables the practitioner to relax and experience quieter and more organised levels of awareness. Scientific studies have shown that people who practise this technique generally display lower blood pressure, fewer heart diseases, a better overall health, fewer signs of ageing and increased levels of creativity. Marvellous changes can also occur when a group of people meditate together: crime, stress levels and violence diminish. In South Africa, school pupils from Alexandra found that their achievements and interpersonal behaviour improved noticeably when they started practising the technique. I had been practising meditation for a few years by then, and Derik had learned the technique a few months earlier. We therefore knew that a restaurant that was inspired by TM would be a special experience.

The restaurant was built in the shape of a double-storey house with a high-pitched roof. It had a wide veranda that ran all along the outside of the upper floor. There was a cool fountain in the garden, and at the side of the house a shiny clean staircase made from dark wood led to the top. We were courteously requested to take off our dusty shoes and socks before walking up the staircase.

We decided to sit outside, where the veranda presented an exquisite view of the garden. That is where we spent the rest of the evening in soft chairs, enjoying a delectable meal and singular communion. Chilled coconut milk for starters, followed by a green curry for Derik and a vegetable breyani for me, topped off with citrus honey ice cream and ginger tea for desert. It was a typical selection of food in the restaurants of northern Thailand, along the border with India. The uniqueness of the experience did not lie in the nature or even the presentation of the dishes, nor in the attentive service or the beautiful building and gardens. Rather, it was noticeable in the energy that enfolded us. Everything was softer, friendlier, clearer, cleaner, simpler and more intense – but without any pretence. The day Derik recalled the wonder of that meal while he was experiencing intense pain, I knew that that special evening would never be more than a single thought away.

The two weeks in Thailand felt far longer than fourteen days. By the end of the trip we were ready to return home. We did not know what awaited us, but it did not matter. The moment was sufficient.

4

Pink, White, Green and Deep Purple

Shortly after our return, we went to the doctor in the neighbouring town of Paarl who had given Derik complementary treatment. All his tests indicated that Derik had reason to feel as well as he did.

On the way home, as we drove past the stately old homes in the main street of the town, I had a very clear, deep sensation that everything in our lives was about to change, and that it would all be for the better. Somehow I **knew** that the year 2000 would be the start of a particularly happy period in my life. I shared my revelation with Derik. Every time we drove back from the doctor in Paarl in the months that followed, I felt an exact repetition of the same strong and vivid feeling. And each time I told Derik about it. I knew, unflinchingly, that everything would change, but I had no idea how. I only knew that I was tremendously excited about the change and that it would benefit both of us.

The haematologist in Bellville carefully examined Derik behind a screen in his surgery. I heard him remark how strong and well Derik looked and that it was a pity that the treatment would make him feel ill again. But, according to the doctor, it was the only solution. The bad symptoms usually lasted only for a week or two, after which things would improve again.

And so Derik started injecting himself with high doses of alpha-interferon every day. Almost immediately he began feeling ill – he lost his appetite and energy and displayed symptoms of chronic 'flu. These were common side effects, and we hoped that they would gradually disappear, as was the case with most people who used the treatment. But the symptoms grew worse. Derik's sparkle waned with his holiday tan. He grew whiter, quieter and thinner.

We tried to continue with our daily routine as usual. We now confined our work to regular office hours, started to see family and friends again and also went out by ourselves. But we were not at ease – Derik was not reacting normally to the medication. He began to feel worse and worse. Week after week there were subtle changes in his blood counts, even though they remained within the so-called normal range.

According to the doctor there was no reason for concern. Nevertheless, my level of discomfort grew gradually and steadily until it was unbearable. Our cat sat silently beside Derik for long stretches of time, staring directly at him. It was as if she was aware of something we were unable to see. Now, just as earlier that year, I felt as if we were about to tumble headlong over the edge of a precipice. Something was terribly wrong, and we were at a complete loss as to what to do.

On the last Sunday in October we invited two of our friends, Sandra and Heather, over for dinner. Heather inquired after my visibly controlled inner tenseness. Clearing the table led to a discussion in the kitchen, where I confessed to feeling utterly helpless and that I strongly suspected that there was something seriously wrong with Derik. Despite the doctor's reassurances that everything was fine, I knew that something was amiss, and I did not know what to do. She looked at me quietly and then asked whether I had ever considered asking for assistance.

Help? Who would I ask for help? Could one ask for assistance? Was one allowed to? What now seems ridiculously straightforward was such a strange thought at the time. I honestly had not considered asking for help an option. As with all the previous crises in our life (our initial conflict with each other, the career changes, the knowledge that we could not have children), we had tried to manage this matter on our own. I had simply assumed that we would have to get through this on our own. So, whom could one ask for assistance, I wanted to know. Her reply was to ask God, to send my request out into the universe, my friends, my family, anyone – but I had to ask.

Heather's remark eventually led to a turning point in my life. For the first time ever I realised that asking for help was not a sign of weakness. In the following months, I gradually realised that when I acknowledged that I needed assistance, I also acknowledged the power of those who surrounded me and recognised my connectedness to them. In this way, I would be able to step beyond myself, to open myself up and invite others into my life. It becomes an interchange. By allowing other people to strengthen one, one again finds the energy to strengthen them. And so the passivity of a helpless, isolated situation is transformed into an interactive, participatory process between people. But it took a tremendous amount of courage to admit that I was not strong enough to make it through this experience on my own.

The recognition that I needed help was the first step. The second step was to ask for it. I began by asking for help from God and the universe. Thirdly, I had to believe that if I asked for help, I would receive it. I had to make myself receptive to answers and possible solutions. Every step was difficult in its own way.

Around us life continued as usual. My hands would start shaking during a meeting at work, but I was the only one who noticed. Derik would eat less and grow even quieter, but the people around him would continue to chat merrily. I had acknowledged that we were in need of assistance. I had asked for it. Now I had to wait.

After three months of interferon treatment, it was more than the continual 'flu symptoms that concerned us. In the meanwhile, we had also discovered that the facts that had been given to us by the haematologist did not correspond with what we were learning from other sources. I tested the doctor one more time. He answered my question about the possibility of a transplant by stating with great conviction that there was no bone marrow bank in South Africa, and that the procedures involving donor marrow and the patient's own bone marrow had not yet been used successfully. According to him, there had been a small database at Groote Schuur Hospital in Cape Town, but it was now defunct.

By that time I had already managed to get the contact details for the South African bone marrow registry. It was no longer at Groote Schuur, but still existed and was situated elsewhere in Cape Town. I had further ascertained that this bank was electronically connected to information from around the world. Their donor-search unit therefore had access to millions of registered donors. At about the same time, there was a press release about someone who was collecting money for the database, and there were other media reports about successful transplants at the Constantiaberg Medi-Clinic, also in Cape Town. Two weeks after asking for help, my mother gave me a newspaper cutting about an interview with someone who had been treated successfully. Her physician had also given her the name of the specialist. Our trust in the haematologist was, to say the least, shattered.

From Derik's diary:
November 1998

At the beginning of November, I noticed that the leukocyte counts were all nudging in the wrong direction. Despite all my concerns, the haematologist said that everything was normal. (I suspect that he looked at each week's results in isolation, and did not look at the whole picture or at possible tendencies, as I was doing.) That, combined with a few other incidents, caused me to lose my faith in him. I went to a Prof J for a second opinion. Within a few minutes, he had laid all the options on the table and, for the first time, I could make an informed decision. Inter alia, he noted that the prognosis for full recovery was about 70% if I were to decide on a bone marrow transplant, even if it was from a non-related donor – in contrast to the previous quack who had told me that the prognosis was 40% on any treatment, and that I should not consider a transplant because Riekie's blood was not compatible with mine. That was Friday, November 20.

On Monday, 23 November, I had my blood tested as usual. The pathologist was fairly concerned by the results. The previous quack (the haematologist) called me at home at 18:00 and asked me to come and see him urgently at his surgery in the morning. I was going to do that in any case, since I was about to fire him! When I arrived there on Tuesday afternoon, he looked like an undertaker. He told me that I had gone directly from the chronic to the acute phase. (Normally, the chronic phase lasts about three years, the blast phase one year, and the acute phase a few weeks.)

I got the impression that it was truly difficult for him to convey this news to me. He was most astonished when I was not surprised and when I told him that I had in the meanwhile done my own research and had gone for a second opinion. He was even more surprised when I referred to the 70% chance of recovery. He was very unsure of himself and remarked that the advance must have been extremely rapid recently, since when he had last enquired, the results with non-related donors were still very dicey. I should have asked him in which year he had last enquired!

Derik was extremely upset when he telephoned me at work with this news. It was only seven months since we had heard that he was suffering from chronic myeloid leukaemia! When I heard the news, I gasped and began to speak so haltingly that my colleagues immediately ran over to my desk. Their closeness at that moment touched me deeply. We cried over the news together. The haematologist had wanted Derik to go to hospital directly from the surgery – this after he had had the results for more than a day! Derik could not face doing that. He told me that he was first going home. I also packed the things on my desk immediately and drove home to Stellenbosch.

Our home in Paradyskloof was always a place where we could relax completely. The house is built around a living area with a high ceiling, with verandas to the north and the south. It is extremely private and allows one to open the doors wide and still remain completely secluded from the outside world. Derik felt an intense desire to be at home before he went to the hospital. We left only later that afternoon. Neither of us expected him to be coming home again. He did not know that I saw him first walking through the garden saying goodbye to Katerina, our black cat.

From his diary:
November 1998 (continued)
They wanted to send me straight to hospital, but when Marthie and I arrived there, we heard that they would only start the tests the following morning. I immediately negotiated rather to be admitted the following morning, and fortunately,

the sister agreed. That gave us the opportunity to return home and enjoy dinner at De Ouwe Werf on Tuesday evening – ostrich fillet and a toast to my health with my favourite sparkling.

Before dawn on Wednesday morning, the two of us left for the C-clinic in Plumstead – just past Wynberg, towards Muizenberg. When we arrived at the hospital, they drew litres of blood. It felt as if Dracula had attacked me. A bone marrow biopsy and a lumbar puncture lay ahead of me. In the meanwhile, they inserted a "J-line" into me under anaesthetic. It is like a drip, except that the pipe is inserted into my chest, from where it runs under my skin to the main artery in my neck and is connected there. Any form of chemotherapy, antibiotics, blood sampling, etc. is now done through the pipes that were connected to the J-line on the outside of my chest. I have to admit that it is quite comfortable and without pain or discomfort – except for the drip stand filled with fluids that I have to drag around with me at all times. I soon got used to the trolley standing outside the shower while I danced around under the water with the connecting tube, trying to get wet all over!

The results of the tests confirmed that I already had 58% blast cells in my blood vessels. The norm for diagnosing the acute phase is 30% or higher. As if this was not sufficient, the professor then discovered that all "normal leukaemia people" also tend to develop problems with either the myeloid stem cells or the lymph stem cells. It appears I grew up with the notion that if something is worth doing, it is worth doing well, for I had complications with both kinds of cells.

On Friday, the professor started a 7-day, 24-hour course of chemotherapy – which stopped on 4 December. As a result of the chemotherapy, my platelet count dropped to 11 (normal = 140–4200), my haemoglobin to 8 (normal = 12,5–

17,3) and the leukocyte count to 0,4 (normal = 4–11). Two platelet transfers pushed the count up to 63, and after four litres of blood, my haemoglobin was 10,2. I'm also receiving protein, calcium and magnesium supplements in addition to my antibiotics. This all happens via the J-line.

Although the counts look really bad, I am optimistic, for it means that the chemotherapy is working. It's possible that I might be able to go home for seven days sometime later this week. Then it will be back to hospital for a second course of chemotherapy, before a third and last round of the same 7-day, 24-hour procedure. The main aim is to stabilise my blood counts. According to the prof, one can buy time in this way while they look for a suitable non-related donor!

When Derik was hospitalised, we knew that people with CML could be cured by bone marrow transplants. But we did not know whether people with acute myeloid leukaemia (AML) could receive bone marrow transplants. Thus, when we had sat down to dinner in De Ouwe Werf the night before he went to hospital, we had thought that it would be our last meal together. It was an extraordinary evening for the two of us. The food and the service were exquisite. We were blessed to be able to speak about our lives together and about life in general. Contrary to my nature, I was calm and peaceful. The evening was undoubtedly a celebration of life and our love for each other.

The following morning, we waited in Derik's hospital room to hear the doctor's recommendations. We did not think that there was any hope left. The friendly man with his forthright manner and short, stubbled grey hair informed us what the procedure would be – the first chemotherapy session in the hospital would be followed by two more sessions of a week each, followed by three weeks at home, then chemotherapy and radiation and, finally, the transplant. This would mean six weeks in hospital. The whole process would take more or less six months. And yes, Derik still had a seventy per cent chance of full recovery!

In the meantime Derik tried to make himself as comfortable as possible in the hospital and spent his days as constructively as he could.

From his diary:

November–December 1998 (continued)

The isolation unit in which I currently am consists of eight private rooms, each with its own bathroom – every patient must keep his or her germs to him/herself. Normally, there are four sisters on duty for the day shift, and two for the night shift. Every three hours they monitor our temperature, pulse and blood pressure – here nothing happens by chance. I must confess that I'm very fortunate that I haven't yet experienced any side effects from the chemotherapy. I'm not feeling nauseous, but my hair is slowly getting thinner. Yesterday, Marthie shaved it with a number two, and if I was famous enough, I could possibly have started a new fashion trend.

Last Monday, I went through a terrible emotional dip, until I consciously decided to distinguish between who I am and what my blood is. Therefore, if anyone now asks me how I am, I can in all honesty state that I'm fine, but that my blood is not doing well. I also asked Marthie to bring me a picture that was taken during the Two Oceans marathon. I realised that I had started another marathon – the principle is exactly the same. Sometimes everything goes well, sometimes less so. At times I feel tired, then I want to walk rather than run. The most important thing is to complete the marathon. And that is definitely my only goal here – to leave here healthy!

I asked for my computer, as well as books on France, Mexico, feng shui, reflexology, astrology, Chinese and Indian medicine, ancient church history, two leisure books and the Bible. Now I really have the time to read everything that has always interested me, but which I have never had the time for. I also have time to do some introspection and to philosophise about the meaning of life and "work". I have discovered that I wish to live, not because I fear death, but because I enjoy living, and because there are still so many things and places I would like to investigate and experience. This is in glaring contrast with how I felt when I was admitted under the impression that I only had a few weeks left! This decision has helped me to get up at six every morning, do my exercises, shower and get ready for breakfast. The rest of the day I spend effectively doing research (I have always wanted to write a story), listening to CDs and, every now and then, watching the 'Boks playing really awful rugby and cricket!

But surely this is enough about me for now. Remember that I am in solitary confinement in a room measuring 3m x 4m.

The hospital was about a forty-minute drive from our home and some twenty minutes away from where I was then working in Pinelands (at the time, I was the manager of a communication consulting unit with the same firm as Derik worked for). To visit someone at the bone marrow transplant clinic, one first has to ring the buzzer at the entrance to the unit and then ask for permission to visit a particular patient. No one with a sore throat, a cold or any other illness is allowed in. The door is opened to approved visitors only. Once inside, the visitor passes through a sterile cloakroom in which he/she is required to take off his/her shoes and outer clothing. Next, one has to put on clean hospital issue – pink suits for women and green for men, with denim foot coverings. Then visitors have to wash their hands thoroughly, and after a further two doors they are finally inside the clinic.

There is good reason for these precautions. All the patients in the clinic have extremely low leukocyte counts, and thus have very, very little immunity. Those who are being prepared for a bone marrow transplant have no white blood cells, since these cells are consciously and completely destroyed by chemotherapy and radiation. A normal person's body fights thousands of germs, bacteria and viruses daily without the body even being aware of it. But for the patients in this unit, a single germ can result in a serious infection or even death; hence contact with them is limited. Only two visitors are allowed in at a time. One is not allowed to sit on the patient's bed, and even a peck on the cheek is prohibited.

Each unit consists of a "lobby" with a fridge, an exercise bicycle, a work surface, drawers and a basin. This section is used by the nursing staff to store and measure medication. It also serves as a buffer between the patient and the other seven rooms along the hallway. This "lobby" is separated from the main room by a sliding door. The room contains a bed with a light green cover, a bedside table, a painting, a TV against the ceiling, another work surface, a basin and a bathroom. Every room's air is filtered separately, the air conditioning is controlled separately, and all the windows are shut tight.

When I walked into Derik's room on 7 December 1998, I got only as far as the "lobby". He and his drip stand met me at the sliding door. He asked me to wait outside; it was obvious that he had something up his sleeve. I went back into the hall, where I noticed the cleaning trolley next to me. (Every room is washed from top to bottom with antiseptic daily.) I remember being somewhat impressed that despite the priority given to hygiene they still managed to make the cleaning agents smell very pleasant. Then I was ceremoniously invited to enter Derik's room, accompanied by the sound of beautiful string music. The pleasant smell grew stronger. Triumphantly, Derik and his drip stand led me to the cupboard. Inside, nineteen deep purple lavender-scented candles sparkled! My dearest, ever-romantic husband! It was our nineteenth wedding anniversary, and he had got special permission to light the candles for a few moments. As the smoke alarm could be set off, all the candles in their candlesticks had to be in his closet, and he was not allowed to burn them for long.

Suddenly I remembered how one evening, fourteen years before, he had waited for me at our modest little home in Potchefstroom after I had been to a night class. The house was filled with the smell of burned peas, but our living room was ablaze with a mass of lighted candles, and every cushion we possessed was arranged on the floor. Seated on the soft cushions, I was treated to a feast of sausage, mashed potato and second-attempt peas. What a memorable evening that was.

The candles in the cupboard had not been the only surprise of this day. Derik had arranged for a friend to wake me before work. Early in the morning, a very sleepy Pieter had delivered a CD voucher from Derik to our home. His wife Anette was to have brought it over, but she was in labour, and their daughter was born later that morning. (We had heard of Anette's pregnancy on the very day I had told my colleagues about Derik's leukaemia. Now we again shared a special date with Pieter and Anette.)

Later that evening, Derik followed up on the CD voucher, the music, the candles, a hamper and a poem he had written, with nineteen roses and a bottle of Simonsig's special sparkling wine that were delivered by our friend Bart. My dear husband had commandeered a host of people into making it a special day for me!

It was exactly a week after his first session of chemotherapy had been completed. If everything went according to plan, he had to remain in hospital for another week before he could come home and rest for three full weeks!

At this stage, I deliberately did not visit Derik every day. I had very little energy, and tried to spend it as wisely as possible between work, Derik, and my daily chores. My visits to him were alternated with those from friends and colleagues, and occasionally I also went out with them, which helped me to keep a balance.

Thus I went by myself to the wedding of our friends, Tracey and Mark. It was an emotional experience for all of us, since Derik was to have led the service. It felt strange now that he was ill and in hospital. Earlier in the year we had gone canoeing down the Gariep River with Tracey, Mark, Bart and Marjanne, and only three months before we had all gone to Matjiesfontein by train for the weekend. Now, suddenly, Derik could no longer be part of it all.

From Derik's diary:
16 December 1998
Today is the Day of Reconciliation. I rose early and started my daily routine, read for a bit, spent some time on the Internet, listened to Christo and Liesel's CDs and watched TV. Television is such a waste of time. Since I have started watching more television, my creativity has definitely declined and I will have to make use of this time to recondition myself to watch only quality shows. Perhaps I should cancel the M-Net subscription when I get home again.

17 December 1998
Felt a bit lazy about getting up early. They took some blood at half past nine and after that I got moving on my normal

routine. Although I am not showing any external symptoms, I'm feeling tired today and it seems as if the blood in my body is seething. Prof visits and tells me that my bone marrow needs to be stimulated so that he can see whether he can get me out of the unit before Christmas. My white blood count has dropped to 0,3 and my platelets to 11, while my haemoglobin is still 10,5. So, that means a few more days here before I can go home. What do I think? How do I feel? Disappointed? Scared? I feel nothing, because, as usual, I'm suppressing my emotions. Later in the day I realised that I am now in the marathon. There are only two choices – carry on or give up. There is no more bravado that I am **going** to run a marathon, or the conscious self-assurance that I **will** complete the marathon. Now there is doubt – am I capable of completing it? What are the odds against me?

I spent the rest of the day trying to get to grips with the finer details of Microsoft Office, spending some **wonderful** time with Marthie and reading the book, *Healing touch*, that Linda lent me. During the late afternoon and evening, I played with Microsoft's Encarta World Atlas that Pierre had brought on Myrtle's behalf. Once more, I slept like a log!

18 December 1998
Woke up shortly after five this morning, meditated, visualised (only genetically healthily programmed pluripotential cells are allowed to form in my body) and thought about the uncertainty. In my mind, I realised that I was at one of the marathon's water stations. I am tired and less motivated than before, so that giving up has actually even become a thought. I realise that no one else can motivate me, so I get up, ride the bike for 25 minutes and read the book, *Why people don't heal and how they can*. Marthie brought it yesterday – a gift from Henk. Fascinating! Afterwards, I did some stretches, exercised my limp stomach muscles, showered, shaved

and enjoyed a hearty breakfast. I have regained my energy and I know that I will complete the marathon. **I am in control once more and I am not a victim of my blood!!** During the day, I received a leukocyte transfusion and was warned that typical 'flu symptoms might occur.

I ended the day utterly frustrated after surfing the 'Net to find and download more channels and subscriptions. Only junk out there. Watched two Bruce Willis movies and felt quite nihilistic afterwards.

19 December 1998
Woke up at four this morning still feeling very sleepy, but couldn't get to sleep again. At five o'clock A (a sister) waltzed in and was very chatty during her observations, while I felt as if I had woken up on one of Stellenbosch's refuse sites. The glands in my throat are particularly sensitive, and my palate is swollen (especially where I had the abscess after my tooth was filled four years ago). I still maintain that that is when my body started going downhill. That was also when I was working as regional manager, and had run the Comrades. After that, I took part in the Old Mutual Marathon and I couldn't even qualify for the Two Oceans.

After lunch I decided to do something active, so I immediately started cycling, showered, washed my remaining hair (it looks like autumn around me – hair dropping everywhere!) and cleaned my mouth. As a result of the nasal drip in the back of my throat, one nostril is raw down to the septum. I doctor myself with Marthie's wheatgerm oil. It worked well on the sores on my lips.

I realised today that I have suppressed everything I have enjoyed until now. For the sake of survival, I have occupied myself with the here and now. I realise that I miss you terribly, my dearest wife – your presence, your body heat, the feel of your skin against mine, your being with me. Tears well up in my eyes every time I think of you. Maybe I am just being too emotional – I miss Dad and Alta who also went through this experience. How differently I would have dealt with the situation – or would I have? I miss the sun on my skin, the fresh fruit and vegetables we rediscovered in Thailand, I miss the mountains and the feeling of being outside, I miss all the family and friends who support us so much now, I miss the smell of the earth, flowers, and trees, I miss our house, swimming pool and, of course, the other darling little cat! I miss running along the Blaauwklippen Road and the mountain trail, flying, diving, laughing!

Every time my body reacts differently to what I'm used to, I realise that I wonder about the implications. Am I strong enough for this marathon? Will I have enough energy and willpower to complete it? Sometimes, my bravado is very shallow, but I have to keep it up. I cannot afford to wonder about things that are beyond my control. Focus on every day and make it a pleasure so that there is something to look forward to each day.

20 December 1998
As of Tuesday, my fever has been see-sawing and my glands and my gums have become extremely sensitive. I have also developed a sensitivity in my nose that I simply put down to a pimple. This "pimple" erupted on Friday night, caused a secondary infection and by yesterday had eaten through my skin and flesh to the cartilage of my nose. It is a raw, open sore. When I got up yesterday, my glands were swollen as if I had the mumps and I am emotional, irritated and agitated as never before. My dear wife, you had specially arrived early so that you could spend the whole day with me. And how you paid for it!

The telephone is also frustrating me. People call me at all hours of the day and night, whenever it suits them. It's intruding into my privacy, and every time it rings, I can feel my aggression rise. I know they mean well, but they don't realise how much it demands from me to repeat the same information time and again. In any case, I do not really achieve a catharsis by talking. My healing has to come from inside. I unplugged the telephone for the rest of the day and switched my cellphone off.

In the meantime, I've been given an antibacterial ointment to put on the "wound" and at least my glands are less swollen today. My palate is still so sensitive that I can hardly eat. The prof is trying his best to get me home before Christmas. With this temporary setback, that seems unlikely now. I am preparing myself to spend Christmas here, rather than the other way round.

During Derik's first session of chemotherapy, he told me about an experience he had had during the night. I call it an experience, because he says it was not a dream, but an "experience" he had in his sleep. He "woke up" to find an erstwhile conductor of the Free State brass band standing beside his bed (Derik had been a trombone player in this band during his school days). This was strange, as Mr van Woerkom and his wife had passed away many years before. Mr van Woerkom asked him where he was going.

"Home," Derik answered.

The man wanted to know more: "Which home are you going to?" he asked.

To which Derik replied: "To our home in Paradyskloof, Stellenbosch, of course."

Derik's story made me feel content – I felt it was a good sign.

The images of water I had been seeing in my dreams since the start of the year continued, but my excitement about the future also continued. From my office in Pinelands, I sent an e-mail to Derik at his computer in the hospital room:

—— Original Message ——
From: Momberg Marthie
Sent: 20 December 1998 08:55 AM
To: Momberg Derik
Subject: I hope you get it!

My darling
The waters may not be so bright right now
But remember that both of us can swim well
We will get through these waves
It will be a good year
MM

By this time I understood that the water in my dreams contained a message of change. From the dreams it became clear that the water was very powerful and dangerous, but that it would not engulf us. With Derik's help I had always paid attention to my dreams and knew that they usually contained a message I should take note of. Although the dreams predicted great change and potential danger, they increasingly pointed to the start of a new phase and to survival. For instance, I would see the waves breaking as they washed over me, but I would remain standing. The dreams that initially terrified me now filled me with a combination of trepidation and wonder.

From Derik's diary:
21 December 1998
It was a quiet day. I feel much better than yesterday. The antibacterial ointment has really helped.

I am not losing courage. I do get scared (especially after yesterday) when I see how easily my body reacts negatively, since I'm not used to it leaving me in the lurch like that. I have been fortunate until now that I've been able to remain the master of my body through reasonable intellectual control. Now I have been reduced to playing host to other people's platelets, red blood cells and leukocytes in order to stay alive. Until my bone marrow starts producing sufficient leukocytes, I am on a permanent antibiotic drip that performs the function of the white blood cells (it offers immunity).

I have also realised that I've developed a fear of the night. I almost put off going to sleep. Is this because I fear not waking up again once I go to sleep? Or is it the Lasiks that forces me to go to the bathroom every two hours?

22 December 1998
I woke this morning feeling more like my old self, even human. Can once again face the challenges and feel very strong and motivated and all that. My love, your visit was very nice. I remain worried that you are not eating properly and that you're not getting enough rest. You are such a wonderful person with so many talents.

Everyone that visited Derik commented on how much he inspired them. Despite his circumstances, he was still interested in the welfare of others. He never gave anyone any reason to pity him. When visitors entered his room, he was the person they had always known – warm and interested. Even the nursing staff clung to his words. Once, he stood in front of the room's whiteboard in his blue gown, drip stand on the side, and gave a full lecture on the influence of various behavioural patterns on the interaction between team members in the work context. He had a lengthy conversation on the haematological distinctions of the different types of leukaemia with Professor J. and Derik did not try to keep up a front. He was genuinely interested in the people around him. His warmth reflected his passion for life and his fellow human beings. Nevertheless, he did not hesitate to delineate the boundaries when it was in his best interest, and that is why he often did not answer the telephone when he did not feel up to it.

It was during this time in hospital that Derik finally managed to draw a framework of the manuscript he had been thinking about for months on the whiteboard. His book would be about the relationship between various world powers and inventions through the ages, and the way in which groups and individuals have and do use and misuse this knowledge in the name of power. His chart combined thought patterns from divergent concepts into a fascinating whole.

He also designed dresses for me – all of them with a low neckline, either front or back. I could not help but smile at this, as for weeks I had been visiting him dressed in the neatly ironed unisex hospital outfit and denim foot coverings.

It was now shortly before Christmas. During the preceding weeks, we had initially thought that Derik would never return home from the hospital again. Then we had received the wonderful news that there was a possibility of a cure, and we had hoped that he would be home within a few weeks. But now, what should have taken four weeks, had already taken five weeks, and Christmas was around the corner. Derik's infection was still not under control. We desperately wanted him to be discharged, but we also knew the risk would be too big if he was not ready. His leukocyte count first had to reach an acceptable level.

Nevertheless, I had every corner of the house cleaned in preparation. I fumigated the house and disinfected all the curtains, bed covers, carpets and windows in order to create an environment that was as sterile as possible so that he would not be exposed to any infection.

I was still exhausted and felt as if I had no energy. I was also drained by the uncertainty of not knowing what to prepare myself for – would we be together for Christmas, for instance? But on the afternoon of 23 December, I made a conscious decision to prepare everything as if Derik was indeed coming home. I somehow managed to scrape together an enormous amount of energy and by six the next morning I was mowing the lawn. By nine, I was already on my way home from Woolworths with all my shopping, and I made the house look pretty with flowers and decorations. So when Derik telephoned me later in the morning to say I could come and fetch him, my heart rejoiced!

It sounds trite to say that I could not have wished for a better Christmas present. But that is the truth. It was Christmas Eve, and my husband was home – our hope had not failed us. My mother came over, we played Christmas carols and Derik strung dainty white lights across the edge of the veranda next to the swimming pool. I prepared a Christmas dinner in which I tried to follow the hospital regulations, in addition to satisfying Derik's desire for fresh, wholesome food and everyone's expectations of a festive meal. We set the table on the veranda, bathed and dressed for dinner. Derik wore the golden tailor made silk shirt from Thailand. Shortly before dinner, Johann, our general practitioner and friend, popped in, and Bart and Marjanne came over for drinks.

The joy that literally bubbled out of Derik, the ceremonial way in which he poured our wine, the grace with which he moved about in his golden shirt and with his clean-shaven head, as well as the genuine delight he took in the food, touched us all. It was a joyous evening in which we celebrated life and Life.

As was our custom, we exchanged gifts on Christmas Eve. I gave Derik a delicate crystal that had been cut especially for Christmas 1998. He surprised me once again. One of his network of "agents" outside the hospital, this time Johann, had arranged my gift – a paper-thin porcelain bowl by Catherine Glenday. Catherine had engraved the title, "Keeping the ants at bay", on the bottom of the bowl to complement her illustrations. Derik thought the design was remarkably appropriate for his scurrying wife! No wonder Johann had come to "visit" just before dinner! We also lit the chunky round white candle with three wicks – for love, hope and faith – which had been a present from our friend Sandra.

On Christmas morning, my mother and I went to church. It was too dangerous for Derik to be in a large crowd of people, so he stayed at home. In the church, I felt the last bit of energy seeping from my limbs. It felt as if my cheeks were dragging on the ground. I was literally too tired to sit upright or to sing. Back at home, I cried despondently. I was so ashamed of myself. Here my husband was, at home, and the doctor was optimistic that he would recover completely. Why could I not enjoy it too? Despite his serious illness, my husband was sparkling and I, the healthy one, felt as if I was about to drop down onto the floor!

Fortunately my mother was there to help prepare the lunch, or I would not have managed. Derik made me sit down and tried to convince me that something was wrong with me. He insisted that I also go and see the professor, as he was sure that there was something wrong with my blood. Derik felt that my chronic lack of iron was making me feel extremely weak, and he thought that someone could help me. He forced me to make an appointment. Of course, I was terribly embarrassed. What would it look like if I too went to the doctor saying that I also needed some attention?

Two days after Christmas, we returned to the hospital for follow-up blood tests and a routine cleaning of Derik's J-line. The sister came to us in the reception area where we were waiting for the results.

"I have bad news," she said, "the blast cells are back in your blood."

This meant that the chemotherapy had not been successful. He could not stay at home any longer, and had to go back to hospital immediately.

To this Derik replied: "I thought so."

5

The "Blue" Chemotherapy

This was the start of the "blue" chemotherapy. The therapy that was normally used to treat acute leukaemia had not had the desired effect on Derik. He needed to be treated with something much more potent.

A bag filled with a bright blue liquid was attached to the drip and its contents flowed into his veins day and night, seven days a week. Under normal circumstances, this extremely poisonous cocktail was used only in combination with radiation when the patient's bone marrow had to be totally destroyed immediately before the transplant. Since the cocktail is so toxic, it breaks the immune system down completely. Combined with the extremely low leukocyte counts (at times, Derik's counts dropped to 0,01), it was a very, very risky procedure. Infection could very easily occur. But it was the only option. If he went into remission after the second session of chemotherapy, he still had to endure two more follow-up courses before the doctors could do a transplant. That is what the doctor explained to me when I visited him a few days later at the beginning of January.

After he had examined me and taken blood samples, we spoke about Derik. Prof J was as direct as ever. He wanted to know how I felt about Derik's situation.

"It's just a process we have to go through," I replied.

I was not in the least bit anxious. In fact, we were deeply grateful that there was even a chance that he could recover completely. This was more than the previous haematologist had offered us, and moreover, it was obvious that this unit's staff knew what they were doing. We were impressed by the way in which the administrative personnel, the doctors, the nursing staff, the pharmacist, dietician and other specialists worked together as a team and used their collective experience to provide the best service possible. Prof J was regarded as an international expert on leukaemia, and his transplant record was one of the best in the world. Most of all, we experienced warmth and empathy from the entire staff. In this clinic, patients and their families remained people, and were not treated merely as numbers.

But I was not prepared for his reply to my second question: "What if the second round of chemotherapy doesn't work?" The doctor calmly replied that the disease would then take its course and that Derik would die. I remained sitting there with a straight face and showed little apparent reaction. However, later that afternoon when I arrived at the gym in Stellenbosch where I did water aerobics, I started to cry when my fellow swimmers enquired about Derik.

With regard to my condition, during his rounds that evening, Professor J told Derik that his wife was "as anaemic as hell!" According to the test results, my haemoglobin, ferotin, and iron levels were abnormally low. The good news was that he would be able to help me.

Normally only the first session of chemotherapy is administered in the isolation unit. Derik was therefore admitted to the neighbouring haematology ward. Here he had less privacy.

Once again, the medication suppressed his resistance. This was a normal part of the process. For a whole week, the blue liquid in the bag on the drip would flow through his J-line and blend with his blood, but after that, he could return home for three weeks.

Since there was contact between the people in the general ward, we became aware of the other patients, each with his or her own story and personal process. Some of them had already had transplants. We met Wouter, a Grade 10 pupil, and Nico, a friend of mutual friends. Both were being treated for lymphatic cancer. Wouter was still receiving chemotherapy and Nico was being prepared for a transplant. Wouter's sister was going to be his donor, and Nico was fortunate enough to be using his own bone marrow. We knew that there was a seventy per cent chance of survival after a bone marrow transplant. Who would live and who would die? Many patients do not even make it to the stage where they can receive a transplant, because they contract infections and die before this.

Everything went according to plan for Derik, and a week later he was discharged so that he could spend three wonderful weeks recovering at home. But alas, once again his discharge was short-lived. After only three days, he developed a fever. It was ten o'clock at night, and according to the hospital, we had to wait for two hours and then take his temperature again. If it stayed above 37 degrees, he would have to be admitted again. Two hours later we left in a hurry.

And so it happened that Derik, our good friend Hans and I came to be sitting bolt upright in the middle of the night early in January, watching the night nurse – the feverish Derik on his hospital bed, and Hans and I in chairs on either side of the bed. The nurse had to fill in Derik's admission forms. We were all slightly disoriented, some perhaps more so than others.

"What are your symptoms? Do you have any valuables?" she asked the routine questions. "Do you have any allergies? Are you having your period?"

We thought she was joking.

"No," Derik replied courteously, yet tongue-in-cheek. It was kind of the nurse to joke – we were probably looking somewhat tense.

"Are you pregnant?"

The three of us stared at her in stunned disbelief. It was now apparent that she was serious. She repeated the question. She wanted to know whether Derik was pregnant. Good heavens! (I'm still not sure whether she ever realised why we were laughing so much.)

Thankfully, they decided to move him to the isolation ward the following morning. Because of his fever, it was too dangerous to leave him in the general ward. Once more, I took everything I could to the hospital to make his stay there more comfortable: his books, favourite CDs, his computer, pen and paper for taking notes, his marathon photographs, an enlargement of a photograph taken of me in Utrecht and also the letters he had written to me while I was studying there.

Even here in the isolation ward, where no contact between patients was allowed, one gradually became aware of the fact that each of the eight rooms in the unit had its own tale to tell. In the dressing room during the ritual changing of clothes, I sometimes spoke to the relatives of other patients, and Derik also occasionally met other patients in the hallway.

—— Original Message ——
From: Derik Momberg
Sent: Wednesday, 6 January 1999 10:59 AM
To: Friends
Subject: A mere moment

Dear Friends
Thank you for the many messages I have received thus far from all of you. I will respond to each one individually – at least I have time!

Attached is a moment in time that touched me and I would like to share it with you.

A mere moment

I'm in a new room that looks out over Table Mountain – Lion's Head, to be more specific. Today is yet another perfect Cape Town day. I gaze at the clear blue sky and the green lawns outside. Further out, the layers of green range from a yellowish colour to a deep blue-green.

In the park there are two (no, actually three) miniature ducks and four guinea fowl. One of the guinea fowl has four little ones and I'm marvelling at the mother's concern over her young ones. Like all chicks (and children) they start scratching and feeding here and there, and before they know it, they are way out of Mother's sight. Then follows a loud whistling and flapping of wings as the mother draws her chicks in and restores order.

I met another mother here at the BMTU (bone marrow transplant unit) who had brought her daughter down from the Transkei. Every day, she watched warily over her twelve-year-old daughter after the transplant. The daughter's room was next to mine. When the girl arrived here, she was already very weak, but youth was on her side, and she bounced back to life so quickly that it astounded everyone.

Five days ago, both of us independently developed a fever that simply wouldn't break. Mine broke three days ago, but hers kept returning. Just yesterday, I met her and her mother in the passage while they were on their way to the bathroom, and I wished them an enjoyable bath.

Last night, one of the nurses told me that she had spoken to the woman about when the little girl could possibly go home. She was getting stronger every day – except for the fever. The mother was quick to tell her that her daughter still had to get much better. Once the girl was discharged from the hospital, they would have to travel back home by bus or by taxi – a three-day journey. They only had enough money to pay for a bus; a plane ticket was beyond their means. With my philanthropic tendency, I was already trying to find ways in which I could procure aeroplane tickets for them. No patient is supposed to make use of any form of public transport for at least six months after being discharged because of the risk of infection.

At the same time, the nurse told me how the girl had filled in a "Reach for your Dream" form the day before. Since the family doesn't have any money for tickets, the nurse (and I, of course) had hoped that the daughter's dream would be to get two tickets to the Transkei. Her dreams were: 1) to be able to stand on Table Mountain, and 2) to be without pain. During the night, her fever grew worse, and this morning at half past eight, her second dream was realised when she passed away.

PS: As I'm sending you this e-mail, the hospital is still trying to get hold of her mother. She is somewhere in Khayelitsha where she had arranged to stay while her daughter was in hospital.

Some of the patients were strong and energetic after their chemotherapy and the subsequent transplant. Others died – often suddenly, without any visible signs of deterioration. Sometimes, I would see one of the sisters with tears in her eyes, or hear family members crying in the passage or see a lifeless body being wheeled through the double doors of the unit. Late one Saturday afternoon I was on my way home when I passed the professor, his eyes filled with tears after the unexpected passing of a patient.

We were intensely aware of the brittle balance between life and death.

En route to Derik's room, I sometimes saw patients in the passage, on their way to either the theatre or the X-ray division. Some of them were emaciated, with sunken eyes and an expression of despair. It tore at my heart. I was thankful that Derik did not look like that. He was thin, but not emaciated. His head was bald, but there was some sparkle in his eyes, even though we did not know whether the chemotherapy would be successful this time.

Unlike the first time, Derik's body now reacted dramatically to the "blue" chemotherapy. Within a few days, he became a being who was fighting for his life. He struggled to get out of bed to go the bathroom. Any other activity, such as reading, writing or listening to music was out of the question. The puzzle I had bought for him lay untouched. Despite his incredible self-discipline, he struggled to eat, and he lost weight rapidly. The piece quoted above was the last bit of writing he did on his computer while in hospital. He never completed his diary.

The chemotherapy was intended to keep his white blood count low, yet at the same time Derik needed white blood cells to protect him from infections. It was a cruel cycle for, as a result of the lack of leukocytes, his body did not have any immunity. He became ill more easily, and it was more difficult for him to recover. Since the normal activity of his bone marrow was still being suppressed by the chemotherapy, and therefore could not produce enough healthy blood corpuscles, his red blood cells and platelet counts were also extremely low. Bi-weekly transfusions did not normalise his counts, but did manage to counter the worst fatigue and internal bleeding.

In addition, he received intravenous vitamins, minerals and antibiotics and had to swallow handfuls of pills during the course of every day. Even the donor blood that kept him alive held a danger. Although all the blood was selected and tested carefully before it was infused into a patient, there was always a risk that the recipient could contract diseases in this way. At the very least, someone whose resistance was as low as Derik's would develop a fever after every blood transfusion because the recipient's body had to fight the foreign elements in the donor's blood.

It is vital to determine the cause of every serious fever. For days, Derik's temperature hovered between 38 and 41 degrees Celsius, and blood was drawn for analysis. This repeated taking of blood made one realise the value of the J-line. It is quite something frequently to part with large quantities of blood for tests and analyses, and to receive litres of blood and intravenous medication for months on end. With the subcutaneous pipe connected to his jugular, there were no needle pricks, blue marks, painful veins, bandages or the continual search for suitable veins.

We had to wait patiently for the results of the blood tests. One after the other the results came back negative. Something had caused the infection, but what? The longer it took to find an answer, the weaker Derik became, and the more difficult it was for him to react to the medication. We simply had to know what was causing the high fever.

The infection was accompanied by a severe cold fever that made his whole body shudder, even under layers and layers of bedding. At one point, I brought him a woollen cap, but nothing could ease the cutting cold that chilled him to the bone. Without exception, the cold fever was followed by a high temperature that left him glowing with heat. If he was lucky, he had a break of a few hours in which his temperature dropped to 38 degrees before the grinding cycle started all over again.

The chemotherapy was life threatening, but it was our only hope. As the heat and cold racked his body, I kept thinking that it was not only his healthy cells that were being broken down, but that the blue liquid was also attacking the leukaemia cells. It was now or never. The chemotherapy simply had to destroy all the blast cells in Derik's blood and bone marrow.

From one perspective I could look at my sick husband with clinical objectivity and realise that there was a process underway that transcended the visible. When one is in a crisis situation, one does whatever is necessary to survive. This meant that I could not become emotionally involved, but had to channel my emotion into action. I used every available moment to focus my thoughts on how his body was systematically being cleansed of blast cells. I realised that Derik could no longer visualise this for himself because he was too weak. Sitting by his bedside, I therefore prayed over and over again and focused my thoughts on his behalf. Even in my car, shuttling between the hospital, work and home, I tried to destroy the cancer cells in my mind's eye.

I have no idea whether this visualisation helped at all, but at least it made me feel as if I was part of the process. It gave me a focal point and made me goal-oriented. I was therefore able to stand beside him without pitying myself. Derik was running the biggest marathon of his life. He was exposed to extreme temperatures, sweated, thirsted and was in danger of becoming dehydrated. He was suffering severe pain and every single breath took an enormous effort.

From where he lay curled up on his side, he could see all his marathon pictures stuck against the bedside table. He had competed in races because he had enjoyed it, and not because he had wanted to compete with anyone, not even himself. The concepts of winning or losing, even setting a good time, were unimportant to him. His aim was always to **qualify** for the next marathon. He did not want to excel, he did not want to be noticed, he wanted to **experience, to complete and then tackle something bigger.**

Now he was occupied with another race – one that demanded much more than the Comrades. In a manner of speaking, he could no longer "run" during this stage of the race. When all went well on a given day, he barely managed to "walk". Mostly, he told me, he was only "stretching his muscles". It did not feel as if he was covering any ground; he was using all his energy simply to survive the moment. This did not mean that he was passive. He had to ensure that his body was supple enough to be able to walk and run again when the time came to do so. So he kept doing everything he had to – he rinsed his mouth four times a day, he swallowed all his pills, ate his food and drank water. Each one of these activities required an enormous effort on his part, but he did it without complaining, because he understood how important it was within the greater process.

The photographs at his bedside reminded him of the emotions he had experienced during a race – getting tired, wondering whether it was worthwhile, weighing up the options and knowing that one needs clarity about who and what one is and why one is doing certain things. From his experience of running, he knew that these thoughts were a normal part of the process and that a person should not become blinded by the present. Derik had always taught me that one should never fight against the proverbial stream.

"Go with the flow," he would say to me repeatedly over the years when I discussed a problem with him. "Trust the process."

And that was what he was doing now. With brute force he clung to the notion that he was in a marathon. Whether he was walking now, or simply stretching his legs did not matter – he was still in the race. It was all part of the process. He drifted with the stream and trusted that he would reach the shore again. He wanted to complete his race.

I stood beside my husband, but as long as he remained in control of his faculties, I did not want to make his choices for him. I could not run the marathon for him. I could help him, but I could not run for him. He would have to complete the marathon at his own pace and in his own time. Perhaps, under similar circumstances, someone else would have wanted to lean on another person, but that was not Derik's nature. He was inherently independent, and the best thing I could do was to respect that.

Nonetheless, he realised that he needed help. He nominated me as his second, the person who would assist him. I had to stand at the roadside and encourage him on, see to it that he was not dehydrated, give him energy bars at strategic points and every now and then, jog along for company. I had to be at his side for the whole race, also when he crossed the finishing line. That meant that my own strength had to hold until the end of the race. I therefore had to manage my own energy responsibly and see to it that I was available at the appropriate times.

My own treatment could not have occurred at a better time. A week after my medical examination at the beginning of January 1998, I received an intravenous iron transfusion. It is a fairly toxic treatment that needs to be monitored carefully, as it can result in death. My mother came and spent the day at my bedside in the hospital. So there Derik and I were lying in the same hospital under the expert care of the same specialist. Four weeks later, I had much more energy, and from then on I steadily started feeling better. It was wonderful to have enough oxygen in my blood again!

My transfusion took place on a hot summer's day late in January. At the time, Derik had been craving fresh peaches for some time – we usually ate fresh fruit daily, and often our breakfast comprised a fruit salad. However, because of the risk of infection, Derik was not allowed to have fresh fruit. On that particular day, my mother brought him some canned peaches in the hope that he would at least enjoy those. Sadly, they were no substitute for the real thing. When I went to visit Derik after my transfusion, I tried to console him by saying that he would be able to eat some of the next season's fresh fruit.

For a few hours that afternoon his temperature was a blissfully normal – 36,6 degrees. Nevertheless, his body was absolutely defenceless. He was extremely concerned that I wanted to drive back to Stellenbosch on my own after the transfusion. He would have preferred me to have stayed over at my mother's place as she lived closer to the hospital. I therefore promised to give him a call the minute I got home.

Unlike Derik, I did not think twice about the effect the treatment would have on my driving abilities. When I called him from home about three-quarters of an hour later, his temperature had risen to 42 degrees. So delicate was his system that his body had reacted violently to his concern about my driving home. We both got a tremendous fright. The fever lasted a few hours and thankfully broke by about ten that evening. I felt really bad about the effect my thoughtless actions had had on him. This incident showed, yet again, how concretely our bodies react to our emotions.

I very much wanted to help Derik, but I felt that I just was not doing enough. While my husband lay shivering from the fever, I could only stand helplessly by his bedside. I spent hours with him, reading, massaging his feet and visualising his recovery on his behalf. The more time I spent at his bedside, the more my respect for the nursing staff grew. The patience, love and dedication with which they attended to him went beyond professionalism. He received the best possible treatment in the hospital. But nothing the staff did could guarantee that the chemotherapy would destroy all the blast cells, or that the cause of the fever would be discovered. If this infection got the upper hand, Derik's body was too weak to fight it, and he would surely die. Would my visualising be strong enough? Could my love help him? What else could I do?

These thoughts all crossed my mind as I sat in front of my computer at work, helplessly wondering what I could do. Derik was ill, very, very ill. He was too feverish and too weak to think or to make any decision for himself. We were in a wild maelstrom, and I wanted to prevent us from drowning. And then I thought once more about Heather's words. I did not have to achieve everything in my strength alone.

Since I was sitting at my computer, it was not difficult to ask for help. I sent my first e-mail to colleagues who had at some time or another made known their empathy with Derik and me. I now simply pushed my natural shyness aside and expressed my deepest wish to them – some I did not even know very well. They came from different racial, cultural, religious and social backgrounds, but, I argued, they had all said that they were thinking of us. Now I took them up on their words. I requested my colleagues consciously to focus their thoughts, prayers and energy on finding the cause of Derik's fevers so that he could be treated effectively, and so that the blast cells could be destroyed.

The following day we received the results of Derik's latest test. It was positive! Derik's fever had been caused by a tuberculosis bacterium.

Nearly everyone is a carrier of the TB bacterium, but a healthy person's immune system is strong enough to suppress it. However, in extreme cases such as Derik's, the disease is activated. Now that the cause of the fever had been identified, the treatment could begin.

Over and above the TB, one of Derik's shoulders was virtually covered in shingles that ate at his tissue and was spreading rapidly. There were further signs of the tremendous erosion of his body: his right cheek was tightly swollen in the exact place where he had had the tooth attended to a few years earlier. The spot had been bothering him ever since. His stay in the hospital stretched to four, five, six, seven weeks. The follow-up session of chemotherapy was long overdue, but Derik was too sick and too weak to undergo it. His leukocyte count first had to reach normal levels before he could be treated again.

It was now important to me that I spend as much time with him as possible in case he felt like talking, but mostly because my presence calmed him. He did not want to receive any visitors at this time. He purposefully sought silence, and I was his only contact with the outside world. It was a time in which he turned inwards in search of clarity, a time when the outside world was less important. His thoughts centred on the question: "Who is God?" and he also wanted to understand who he was in relation to God.

Day after day I sat quietly beside him. Sometimes, I visualised on his behalf, sometimes I read, worked or simply sat. It was during this time that he gained clarity on the single significant problem in his life. Early one afternoon, after another fever attack, he was resting. After a long time, during which I thought he was sleeping, Derik broke the silence.

"I now know what is happening to me," he said.

It was something he had been aware of for years, but now, for the first time, he saw a real connection between this issue and his illness. When he explained his insight, I cried with relief. I had noticed the smothering effect of this issue on Derik's life over a considerable period of time, but I had been unable to point it out to him. If I had, he would not have reached this insight on his own, and he would probably have continued to suppress and deny his feelings. Moreover, I had not seen the correlation between the problem and the way in which it had manifested itself in his body. Derik decided to tackle the problem head-on. He knew the rhythm of his fever attacks, so he decided that he would telephone the people concerned later that afternoon, when he had another lull.

It was a long telephone call, for which he drew together all his strength. He spoke to the people concerned in an honest, direct, definite, yet tactful and loving way. It gave him an opportunity to face the problem and deal with it, to make peace with it and to forgive. At that moment, I knew clearly and distinctly that the blast cells would disappear from Derik's body, and that he would regain his health fully.

To my mind, this struggle in Derik's life was no bigger than the issues I, and many other people, wrangle with daily. It still amazed me that someone who was so upright and integrated could become as ill as he did. At least, I told myself, all possible emotional stumbling blocks in the path of his recovery had now been removed.

Whether resolving this issue played a role in Derik's physical well-being can, of course, not be determined by conventional medicine, but it is significant that before the discussion he had a high temperature, and that it subsided immediately after the discussion. He also did not have another prolonged bout of fever during this chemotherapy session. Perhaps the medicine was effective, but whatever the reason, he gradually began to feel better. He still had fever attacks, but the intervals between were longer and his temperature no longer exceeded 38 degrees.

We began to breathe more easily again. Derik's condition now improved rapidly. His leukocyte count increased and consequently his body was able to fight the infection. The area affected by shingles started to shrink, his lungs no longer hurt as much and the fever receded until eventually his temperature normalised. The most important thing was that a bone marrow biopsy indicated that all the blast cells had been destroyed!

We were exuberant, even though Derik could come home only for a few days and not for the full three weeks as we had initially hoped. As before, Derik got into the passenger seat of the car. He was weak and his leukocyte count was relatively low, but the sparkle in his being was clearly visible. We could go home together, and he was in remission. At last, he was in remission!

Along with his eagerness to go home, there was also a sense of careful trepidation. He now had to breathe unfiltered air, his body experienced the shift in temperatures from day to night, he was wearing everyday clothes and he felt different textures under the soles of his feet. Suddenly, he was away from the structured, yet safe, environment of the isolation unit. Every object he touched, every hand he shook, held the danger of infection.

Once more, I cleaned every corner of the house. And once more, we carefully followed the prescribed procedures when preparing food: no dish, opened tin, packet or bottle could be kept for more than a day before the contents had to be eaten. No fresh foods such as fruit or salads were allowed – all vegetables had to be peeled and rinsed in sterile water before they were cooked. Some cooking methods, such as stir-frying, were prohibited, as well as foods like muesli, nuts, processed foods, fresh milk and cheese. All his food had to be kept separately. Over and above all this, he had to continue with the multitude of pills and had to take two supplementary liquid meals a day.

After the many weeks of a monotonous pink, green and white existence, the few days at home were almost overwhelming. He noticed every bit of detail – the white rose on the blue tablecloth at our first dinner, the colours of my summer dresses, the different birdcalls. Everything was special to him. It was moving to see how glad Katerina, our cat, was to see Derik again. The fact that she recognised him despite the immense changes he had undergone helped to make Derik feel at home. She followed him everywhere – standing, sitting or lying wherever he went. She guarded him every minute. This time, his recuperation at home was not interrupted by a fever.

The two of us, who had never before celebrated Valentine's Day, spent the evening of Sunday, 14 February, beside the pool. From there we could watch the rose-coloured reflection of the setting sun against the Stellenbosch Mountain. Seven heart-shaped candles in ceramic holders – a gift from a friend – burned along the edges of our table. A few friends came to visit us during the course of the evening. It was Derik's last night at home before he went back to hospital for his third round of chemotherapy.

6

Easter Eggs Filled with Holes

—— Original Message ——
From: Momberg Marthie
Sent: Monday, 15 February 1999 9:08 AM
To: Colleagues and friends
Subject: Good news!

Dear colleagues, friends
Over the past weeks, you have helped me to pray for Derik's recovery. Today, I have good news:
- The origin of the terrible fever has been identified. He now receives the right treatment and the fever is under control.
- His blood is "clean" and he is in temporary remission.
- Derik was at home for a few wonderful days!

Along with all the above good news, the doctor has expressed his concern. Although Derik is in temporary remission, his blood cells are still not forming properly. The third course of chemotherapy that starts today is therefore of utmost importance.

We are very grateful for the good progress, but we realise that there is still a long road ahead. Nonetheless, we are both optimistic that the further treatment will be successful.

Thank you so much for your support.
MM

Almost three months had passed by since Derik was first hospitalised. It was also three months since the professor had launched an international search for a suitable bone marrow donor. At first, the bone marrow registry informed us that there might be a donor in Durban. We were very excited about this, since having a local donor would reduce the cost considerably. Unfortunately, further tests showed that this donor's bone marrow did not match Derik's.

Money was by far not our biggest concern. What was important, was finding a donor whose genetic make-up was as close to Derik's as possible. We were hopeful that a suitable donor would be found somewhere. When I had asked the professor during our first visit to him what the chances were of finding a non-related donor, he had replied: "We have never not found a suitable donor." This was comforting.

In the meantime, our friends and colleagues had also wanted to help. They filled in application forms, spread information about pathologists, explained the process involved to friend and foe alike, and had thus recruited many new donors. It is actually a relatively simple process – one visits a pathologist, fills in a form and has the doctor draw a few vials of blood. There is no cost involved for the donor, as long as he or she is prepared to help anyone anywhere in the world, and not just a particular patient. The other conditions are that the potential donor is healthy and between the ages of sixteen and fifty. Once the blood has been taken, a basic identification of the donor's tissue type is made and this information is then included in an electronic database. Everyone that is included in the database receives a donor card with his or her personal details on it.

Hundreds of thousands of combinations are necessary in order to find a single suitable donor, and the search takes between three and six months. At this stage, there were only about twenty thousand registered donors in South Africa, but the South African Bone Marrow Registry (SABMR) in Cape Town has access to databases in North America and Europe that have details of many more potential donors.

At the start of the search, the registry compiles a shortlist from the database. If it appears that the DNA structure of a donor's bone marrow corresponds with that of the patient, the donor is asked to donate more blood for further, more detailed tests. At this point, the donor may decide to withdraw from the process. Donating bone marrow is almost like donating blood. In fact, the Constantiaberg Medi-Clinic no longer does transplants with bone marrow, but uses blood stem cells.

During the transplant, the stem cells in the patient's bone marrow, which were deliberately destroyed by chemotherapy and radium, are replaced. The donor is connected to a cell separator in which the blood cells are separated, and the stem cells can then be "harvested". Only the stem cells are removed, not the blood. After proper treatment, the stem cells are immediately transplanted into the recipient by means of a process that resembles a blood transfusion. If all goes well, the patient's body accepts the cells and starts to produce healthy red and white blood cells and platelets.

Between 1998 and 1999, this particular clinic had done an average of two transplants per week on adults and children. In contrast to the assurance given to us by Derik's previous doctor, the fact was that these transplants were being done successfully, and that an average of seventy per cent of those who received this treatment recovered completely.

For the third round of chemotherapy, Derik was again admitted to the haematology ward where patients shared rooms. On his left, a woman from the Eastern Cape sat knitting beside her husband's bed. She talked incessantly about how her bathroom floors and her carpets were being damaged by family members who were staying in their house while they were in Cape Town for her husband's treatment. Again and again, she would regale people with the gruesome details of how the damage had occurred. She did not take much notice of her husband, who lay silently staring into space.

The man's temperature was 38 degrees – he thought this was disturbingly high, and he was terrified of contracting further infection. In a rare moment, when his wife had gone for a cup of tea, he spoke up and shared his fears with Derik. He mentioned that he had heard that TB was now "also on the run" in the hospital. Derik tried to set him at ease by telling him about his own experiences with fevers and how they had successfully treated his TB. Unfortunately, it had exactly the opposite effect on the terrified man.

The bag of blue liquid seeped into Derik's veins drop by drop. Another bag filled with fluid and antibiotics was attached to him. We waited patiently for the week to pass. Hopefully, everything would go well this time so that Derik could come home to rest for the full three weeks.

—— Original Message ——
From: Momberg Marthie
Sent: 03 March 1999 02:10 PM
To: Colleagues and friends
Subject: Derik

Dear friends and colleagues
Just a short update on Derik's progress:
After the third chemotherapy session, he came home last week – looking thin and weak, but feeling just fine. Unfortunately he stayed for only five days. The fever returned and I had to take him to the hospital yesterday afternoon. We don't know yet what caused the fever, or how long he will be in hospital. However, we remain positive that he will be

able to come home again before the fourth and final round of chemotherapy.

We hope to find a donor in the near future.

Thank you so much for your continued support. Derik sends his regards and he has asked me to thank all of you – your support and prayers carry us.

Both of us are looking forward to the day that he will be healthy.

MM

Alas, the fever was back. This time Wouter shared the room with him. Derik enjoyed sharing with the teenage boy. It was good to see how well he was doing. Like all the other patients, he had no hair, but otherwise he looked glowingly healthy. The peace that radiated from him struck me every time I saw him. He was remarkably mature for his age. Just like everyone else, he wanted to go home as soon as possible after his chemotherapy, but he did not go on about it or complain loudly as some of the adult patients did after weeks in the hospital. Wouter was receiving his final chemotherapy before his transplant. His treatment, unlike Derik's, had gone smoothly for most of the time.

After work in the evenings, I sat beside my husband. His legs, with their beautiful calves, lay on top of the covers, as red as beets against the white linen. This was the result of the previous round of chemotherapy. Up to now, we had been under the impression that his body had reacted exceptionally and violently to the treatment, but we had no idea of what was in fact possible.

It was early March, but Derik was not sweating as a result of the Cape heat. The room was air-conditioned. The sweat I sponged off his body was caused by a huge infection in his face. The abscess in his tooth that had been bothering him for four years now made the right side of his face swell up to a few times its normal size. His face was distorted. I used lukewarm water to sponge him down, but I could not do it all the time since the evaporation on his skin could cause dehydration. Derik tried to drink small quantities of fruit juice through a straw, but he barely had enough breath to do this. The infection had caused his respiratory tract to become coated with a sticky, transparent mucus. It poured from his nose continually. He had lost all feeling in his upper lip and in the skin above the swelling. He could therefore not feel the fluid running from his nose, and I had to help him clean it.

At the bed next to us, Wouter's father sat peeling peaches for the two of them in the afternoon's twilight. He and his wife took turns to drive through from a neighbouring town to visit their son. Like me, Wouter's father brought work with him – neither of us could afford to neglect our work altogether. Sometimes, Wouter and his mother visited the hospital's coffee shop to have something nice to eat and drink.

Derik found it difficult to move from his bed. His temperature was again hovering between 38 and 41 degrees. The infection in his face made it impossible for him to eat anything. The mucus was no longer clear and was now also blocking his throat. At best, he tried to swallow liquid foods. Initially, he could manage to walk the few steps from his bed to the bathroom by holding onto his drip stand for support. This worked as long as I went ahead quickly and opened the doors for him and then helped him onto the seat. Later, I had to support him as he walked.

A daily bath was still essential, as even the normal peeling of skin on the human body could cause a serious infection. It took the best part of an hour to get through the process, but we both looked forward to it. When the door closed behind us, and the warm water flowed over Derik, I would sink down onto the floor beside him. The seclusion of the bathroom and the sensation of water and silent steam allowed us to escape momentarily from monitors, meters and people. The drip stand with its bags and pipes was still there, but we were almost completely free from the world outside. It was rest and normality in the middle of our tension-filled reality. Then I could touch him in private, and Derik was able to relax in the weightlessness of the water. In these moments, we felt as if we were still ourselves, Derik and Marthie, husband and wife.

The infection in Derik's cheek grew worse, and the professor called in a stomatologist. He decided to do an operation to clean out Derik's sinus passages. The operation was scheduled for a day on which I had to do a presentation for an important client in Durban. I was not sure whether to go on this assignment or not. I discussed the matter with Derik and the specialist. In the end, I decided to make the trip.

I left early in the morning, and put on my most professional face in front of the forty trustees of the retirement fund. After the presentation, I had a friendly chat with the consultants and the actuary, and flew back to Cape Town that same afternoon.

The operation was unsuccessful. The doctor managed to drain a fair amount of fluid and removed the tooth that had been bothering Derik, but he was unable to solve the problem. It was indeed the tooth that had been causing the infection. But the infection had already spread to the surrounding soft tissue and could not be removed surgically or by draining the wound. The surgeon also found that the infection had eaten away the cartilage and the nerves in Derik's cheek. The loss of sensation in his cheek and upper lip would be permanent. Blood tests confirmed that a fungus had started this virulent infection.

Derik's fever increased, and the doctors decided to transfer him to the isolation section of the bone marrow transplant clinic. Not once during the months of his illness had Derik even uttered a complaint. This transfer, however, came as a great relief to him, as well as to me. It meant that he would receive more intensive care, and the greater degree of privacy would give him more personal space. He was now given some extremely strong antibiotics intravenously, and we hoped that this specialised treatment would clear the fungal infection rapidly, as had been the case when he had previously received specific treatment.

But there was no indication of improvement. On the contrary, the infection spread into his respiratory tract and lungs. He could now breathe only through his mouth. His throat was partially blocked by the thick slime and the feeding pipe. He could no longer eat or drink, so they had to insert a pipe through his nose, down his throat and into his stomach so that he could be given liquid meals. Another complication occurred. His sugar levels were too high and he could therefore receive only a particular mixture that was suitable for diabetics.

The physiotherapists and specialists all tried to help him. Many steam treatments, X-rays and three operations followed, but these managed only to relieve the symptoms by sucking out the worst of the mucus. A second tooth was removed. A lung surgeon suggested that he surgically remove the infection from Derik's lungs, but we did not think this was feasible. If even the slightest bit of the fungus remained after the operation, the infection would return.

Derik's weight dropped from 74 kilograms to 56. (When he was healthy, he weighed between 78 and 84 kilograms.) His strength also decreased rapidly. On his own insistence, I now bathed him in his bed daily. Every time one of the sisters wanted to wash him, he told her that his wife would be there soon, and that she would do it. His refusal to have the hospital staff wash him had nothing to do with being shy. Derik had always been one of the first to volunteer for a skinny dip. He had introduced a number of our friends to this practice and his body had glided into the water of many mountain pools throughout the country.

Rather, it was more about the opportunity of being touched in a calming, restful manner. Having a clean skin was a side issue. Our rhythms and our way of doing things were the same, and so washing him in bed gave us both the opportunity to reaffirm the physical bond between us. Four months had already passed since he had been hospitalised. In that time, he had spent only a few days out of the hospital. As we had been used to touching each other all the time, we now leaped at the opportunity offered to us by water and soap. It was good to help him in this way.

The support from colleagues, friends and family that I relied on so unconditionally undoubtedly helped me to sit beside Derik daily without pitying him. Although I consciously chose not to entertain pity, I did experience a superhuman inner energy. I am not a typical motherly, caring person. When I had had to wipe children's noses during my first teaching assignment at a primary school, I had felt very squeamish. Yet I could help my husband with great love and patience. Only the visible parts of his being were affected. That which he truly was, and with which I had fallen in love, was more beautiful and clearly visible than ever before. I could observe Derik's physical decline without becoming distressed about it, since I had never considered his body to be the same as his person. His inner strength, peace, grace and charm were far too strong.

What did distress him, however, was the fact that he had started hallucinating. Dr Derik Momberg, minister of religion, business manager and clinical psychologist, alias "leading psychologist", as one newspaper had referred to him in the late eighties, the person who had helped so many people and who was renowned for his wisdom and realism, no longer knew where reality ended and fantasy began. The hallucinations had a simple explanation – he was suffering from a lack of sodium as a result of dehydration, although we did not realise this immediately.

It was Derik himself who told me about the hallucinations. As time passed, I also became aware of them. They did not occur all the time – only when the delicate balance in his body was disturbed. He described how he would wake up and see children performing forced labour. Day after day he could clearly hear them labouring like slaves, chopping stones with their chisels. (In reality, workmen were doing alterations outside his window, and he was in fact hearing them using their chisels.)

On another occasion he was searching for a tree. If he could find the tree, he would be able to climb it and get out of the hospital. A few days later, he realised that it was an illusion that had him looking for a real tree similar to the one depicted in the painting at the foot of his bed. On yet another occasion, after a steam therapy session, while lying at a slant with his head in a downward position, he asked me whether there was indeed a film being shown in front of him. He described the characters from an espionage story in great detail. These incidents made my heart writhe with anguish. My husband realised that he might be hallucinating, but he was not sure. Yet he still had the courage to try to ascertain whether he was really losing contact with visible reality. He was definitely not going to surrender to his circumstances.

Once he had a truly horrible experience. In front of a nurse who was doing routine monitoring he started saying that he had to get off a bus urgently because someone planned to attack the passengers. It was a very real, intensely threatening experience for him, and I had never heard Derik panic as he did then. He explained his strategy to us with great effort since his throat was so dry that he did not have the full use of his voice and he breathed with difficulty. The other people were fleeing blindly he told us, but he consciously chose to walk calmly so that it did not look as if he was fleeing. Worst of all, he did not know whether he would be able to escape from the danger in time. He was almost hysterical and on the verge of tears. But through it all he retained his inherent politeness and presence of mind. Since the nurse was a foreigner and thus could not understand any Afrikaans, Derik told his story to me bit by bit in Afrikaans before turning to her and repeating what he had said with the same intensity in English. He wanted both of us to understand him perfectly.

At Easter, remembering his magical games in our garden, I bought him a very special Easter egg. It was the same size as the ones of the previous year, but this one was divided into two equal sections, each filled with handmade chocolates. The whole egg was beautifully gift-wrapped in a box with a bow around it. As I gave it to him, he informed me in great earnest that I was supposed to **know** that under no circumstances was he allowed to eat anything with holes in it. So I promised to keep the egg in the fridge until he came home. I did not know whether to laugh or cry, and much later, in a private moment, I did both.

My own dreams about water continued. But now they were all positive.

I dream that we are driving in a rattling old bus with a group of people, travelling through an endless stretch of land. The road runs all the way from the south to the north of the British Isles, except that it does not in any way resemble the typical green landscape. The countryside is extremely barren – littered only with the remains of dried plant material. Ahead of us lies a long, steep hill. Will the ramshackle bus be able to get over the hill? Will we make it? What if the bus breaks down, or something else goes wrong? And yet, after a huge struggle, we do reach the top safely. What a wonderful surprise! From the top of the hill at the northernmost point of the British Isles, we look out on a fertile landscape with tropical vegetation and luxurious wooden huts on stilts in clear water. The sea is filled with multicoloured fish like the ones we saw in the Andaman Sea around Phuket when we had snorkelled there, only bigger and more beautiful. We drive down, and suddenly I find myself in the lukewarm water. I forget about the recent journey as my body glides under the surface of the crystal sea. From under the water, I look up at the wooden huts on their stilts, and also at the rich diversity of sea life that surrounds me. It is an awesome sight.

When I woke up the following morning, I knew that I had to tell Derik about this dream – especially that we would reach such a beautiful destination after all the hardship, and that the water would be crystal clear!

As the chemical balance in Derik's body was restored, his hallucinations diminished. He gradually got better; every day was a step towards normality. One of the specialists suggested that we suck the mucus out of his nose and throat through a plastic pipe. We had to work very carefully to avoid damaging any of Derik's membranes. After we had followed this procedure repeatedly for many days, he was eventually able to breathe through his left nostril. He also started coughing, which helped to get rid of the mass of mucus that had formed in his lungs and his throat. Gradually, the swelling subsided. Eventually, I was able to help him swallow liquids again. It was a tedious and a painful process: a spoonful of water or fruit juice at a time, followed by a fit of coughing and spluttering, then sucking mucus from his mouth and throat, and finally repeating the process until he could endure some moistness on the back of his throat. He was too weak to hold the spoon himself. I would spread the spittoon, tissues, towels, mouthwash, sterilised cotton swabs, the water and the spoon in a circle around us on the bed and the table, and then feed him drop by drop. The nursing staff came to help us remove the mucus at the push of a button. I was elated when he was eventually able to hold down a whole spoonful of liquid and, much later, swallow half a bottle of baby food. As the moisture returned to his throat, his voice also became normal again.

With the help of the physiotherapist and the nurses I encouraged Derik to do simple tasks again. For instance, he had to raise his elbows about thirty centimetres off the bed while he was lying on his back, and practise sitting up for ten minutes a day. One day, when an assistant asked if I would like a cup of tea, Derik casually asked her to bring him one too. The way he said it made it sound like the most natural thing on earth for us to be drinking tea together. He coughed and spluttered his way through half a cup of *rooibos* tea, and all the bedding had to be replaced by the time he had finished, but we understood the significance of his attempting to do an everyday activity with me very well. Derik had held his own cup, and we had had tea together.

And so we progressed until he was able to stand again. Two weeks later, he was able to walk down the passage. Every afternoon, we practised until he was able to complete two lengths of the passage and was strong enough to get into a bath with my help.

As before, I would wash him from head to toe, dry him and put cream on his gaping body. His arms and legs were thin, and his knees and elbows stood out grotesquely. The shoulder on which I had rested my head for years was no more than a sharp piece of bone covered by a thin layer of skin. Even now, I felt as if I was detached from it all. The external change was occurring right before my eyes, and yet it was not. I did not allow what I saw to hurt me. I did not let his physical suffering dictate my feelings. The first time I helped him shower and saw his naked profile through the shower door, he looked even thinner than I had imagined. His body was no more than a skeleton that could tumble over at any time. By contrast, under the stream of water his spirit stood erect and proud. For the first time in three months he had washed himself.

It was easy not to pity Derik, because his behaviour never lent itself to that. His essential being had never been situated in his body. That was merely a form in which his presence was cast. His essence was something much bigger and much deeper. I never thought of him as a patient. Perhaps that is why I never felt the urge to share the specific details of his circumstances with anyone. I respected him immensely for the grace with which he controlled every moment, irrespective of whom or what he was dealing with, despite the circumstances.

It was difficult for him to eat proper food again with two molars missing. The hollow in his cheek where the infection had eaten into his tissue was filled with three metres of antiseptic cord, but the wounds where the teeth had been, lay raw and open. These would recover only once his leukocyte count reached relatively normal levels. I therefore tried to suggest combinations that complied with the hospital regulations, but which he would be able to eat. However, somewhere between what I requested and what the kitchen produced, something always went wrong. Meal after meal arrived with plates piled high with food he was unable to eat. After a while, the kitchen pureed all his food, but this looked so unappetising that Derik stubbornly refused to touch it. Eventually we found a workable solution – for instance, steamed fish with a butter sauce was palatable. Slowly his weight crept up from 56 to 59 kilograms.

By the middle of April, on the day before his mother and sister came from Pretoria to visit him, the swelling in his cheek had receded so much that the raw flesh that had been pushed out of the socket of his right eye for weeks could carefully be put back into place. The eye was neatly closed with a plaster so that what should have been inside would stay there. By this time, the obstruction in his respiratory tract had almost cleared and he could breathe partially through his nose. As far as I was concerned, he looked relatively respectable when he received his first visitors in weeks.

However, his mother and sister were utterly shocked at the extent of his physical deterioration. Although they longed to be with him, they actually saw very little of him. During their five days in Cape Town, they saw him only twice. Derik was still far too weak to receive visitors and five minutes into the first visit he had to be given oxygen as a result of the physical and emotional exertion. He improved daily however, and their second visit lasted fifteen minutes.

During these weeks, I spent every available moment at the hospital. My colleagues were wonderfully supportive. They allowed me to work in the evenings so that I could go to visit Derik early in the morning and again late in the afternoon. Without them, I would not have been able to cope. They did everything possible to make my life easier by generously taking over many of my responsibilities. I will always be indebted to my team members – Charlene, Sue, Janine, Anette and Nikki.

Myrtle, Derik's secretary, kept his colleagues up to date on developments. She diverted calls and visitors and created opportunities for people to show their love and interest by sending us electronic messages and cards. Derik's colleagues even produced a video to convey their "personal" messages. It was another blessing that the hospital was a mere twenty minutes by car from my office in Pinelands.

In addition to these gestures, I will forever remember the support and love I received from our friends, then and later.

When I arrived home at night, totally exhausted, one of the Müllers or a friend from the swimming club would bring me a meal. Bart looked after the maintenance of our house, Deon serviced the pool week after week, Piet and Griet did my chores for me, and Susan and Tjuks embraced my weariness in the comfort of their graceful home during weekends. In between, other friends sent flowers, books, rusks, fruit, music and cards. Ilse compiled an album of photographs and stories. This album was introduced by a quote from DC Brock:

"Friendship is a miraculous happening between people... a warm, intangible understanding that reaches from one to another. Friendship is independent of logic and refuses to be categorised... it is unique, inexpressibly dear and to be cherished. It is a gift freely given."

Each one of them shared what he or she was able to give best. When the telephone kept ringing so often that I was unable to have a bath or eat before ten at night, friends of friends lent me an answering machine. I recorded an account of Derik's condition on it daily, and people accepted that I was unable to return all their calls. The system worked well because it enabled everyone to be updated on Derik's condition and also allowed them to assure me of their presence. In addition to this, Hans and Anneke, and occasionally also Susan and Tjuks, called people on my behalf when I felt that we needed their immediate and urgent prayers and energy.

Perhaps what I valued most was the energy and time our friends and their children, our families, colleagues, neighbours, various congregations and even strangers spent focusing their thoughts and prayers. For months, our friends and family involved their respective prayer and spiritual support groups in the process Derik and I were going through. Week after week they dedicated us to the love and compassion of our common God. In this way we became part of a wide support network that stretched across cultural and religious boundaries. We were no longer alone. We not only learned how to ask for assistance, we also learned how to receive it. We were enclosed by the warmth and all-encompassing love of those who surrounded us.

And all the time Derik kept getting stronger, until he was finally discharged on 19 April. It was roughly a year since he had been diagnosed with chronic myeloid leukaemia. Now all that remained was the fourth and final round of chemotherapy and then the bone marrow transplant. It was exactly six months before 19 October 1999.

7

Antibiotics on an Irrigation Pipe

It was wonderful to be at home together. Derik needed a lot of rest before his body could cope with the last round of chemotherapy – which had to follow soon. He grew stronger every day and continued to put on weight. There was no doubt about his endurance and his desire to recover fully.

Our mothers took turns to stay with us to help prepare three fresh meals a day and do the housework. This enabled me to return to working normal office hours.

On 1 May, only two weeks after his discharge, Derik's sister was to get married in Pretoria. It was impossible for us to attend her wedding, since Derik was not allowed to travel by air, and the twelve-hour journey by car would have been too exhausting. However, I had arranged to attend the wedding of a friend on the same day in Stellenbosch. I had planned to go on my own, but the night before the wedding Derik said that he really wanted to go as well. Neither of us thought that this was impossible, but because of the risk of infection we would have to be very careful that he would not be exposed to a large group of people. The following morning we waited for all the guests to be seated in the Presbyterian Church before we slipped upstairs to the gallery. While the rest of the congregation was singing the closing hymn, we sneaked out again. After the service, Derik remained in the car with the windows closed while I sprinkled confetti on the bridal couple and took photographs.

But it was impossible for him to stay hidden like that. Initially, he just rolled down the window to have a chat, then, before I knew it, he was standing outside the car, chatting. Friends attending the wedding dearly wanted to hug him and talk to him. How special it was to see the person, who a few weeks before had been unable to sit upright and who had had difficulty breathing, now standing among his friends chatting. His clothes hid most of his bony body.

The normality of the sunny autumn day – getting dressed and going to a function where we could celebrate someone else's joy – confirmed for us how much we both were still rooted in this life. The experience of the hospital lay far, far behind us.

During a follow-up visit to the professor and the lung specialist, we ran into an excited Wouter and his dad at the entrance to the hospital.

"I've gained four kilograms!" he beamed.

He looked radiantly healthy and we envied him in a good-natured way. He was very excited as he had just completed his final round of chemotherapy and was at the hospital to receive his transplant.

Derik's future looked less rosy. The infection in his lungs had still not cleared completely. This was bad news. The specialist gave us a choice: Derik could either go back into hospital, or we could arrange for him to be cared for at home.

After all the months in hospital, we felt that there was really only one choice. We asked two of our friends, both qualified nurses, whether they would be prepared to give him his intravenous antibiotics at home every day. On alternate afternoons, Emma and Anneliese came to our house. As with the chemotherapy, Derik had to be given his antibiotics through his J-line twenty-four hours a day.

We did not have a drip stand at home on which to hang the medication, so Derik fashioned a workable contraption out of some irrigation piping and a scrap triangular stand. We wrapped tinfoil around the light-sensitive medication to protect it. Derik dragged the contraption with him wherever he went. The bag had to hang a certain height above his head otherwise there would not be enough pressure to enable the liquid to flow into his body. This meant that he was now largely housebound, but it was still better than being in a hospital bed.

I wanted Derik to go back to the doctor who had given him complementary therapy before he was initially hospitalised. I hoped that he would be able to help Derik get rid of the fungus in his lungs more quickly, or at least help him to build up his immune system again. But Derik felt that he was already receiving the best possible treatment at the hands of extremely competent specialists. As always, we both felt very strongly about our own opinions. Once again, I had to gain clarity within myself about my role. How far did my responsibility stretch? Did I have to drag my husband to the doctor by his collar? Should I try to influence him subtly until he did what I wanted? Or did I simply have to respect his opinion and accept that he was the sole decision maker when it came to matters that concerned his own body?

I knew that dragging him there by the collar would not work. I would not enjoy doing it and, in any event, Derik would not allow it. Subtle manipulation would also not work because it had never been part of our relationship anyway. We had always been direct and honest and did not try to manipulate each other. If I tried something like that now, Derik would see straight through me, and that would give him reason to doubt his trust in me. But should I let him make his own decision when I was convinced that the doctor would be able to help him? I knew that we did not have unlimited time available to us, and that Derik could not receive chemotherapy before the infection had cleared. I chose the latter option.

Freedom of choice was extremely important to Derik, and if I wanted to do what was best for him, I had to comply with his wishes, not my own. This was a very, very difficult decision for me to make, as his life was at stake. It meant that I had to accept yet again that everything was not in my hands. I had to allow Derik to be in control of the process. I could make a reasonable request and set out my argument, but ultimately he had to decide. I therefore accepted his decision not to seek additional help at this point. I had to accept that we had no guarantees about anything. And yet neither of us believed that the antibiotic would not work. It had succeeded in combating the infection every time up to now – it would be effective once more, we believed.

As the hospital insisted, we paid a visit at least once or twice a week so that the staff could test Derik's blood and clean his J-line. Soon after one of these appointments, Derik's mother called me at work. Derik had contracted a fever and had to return to the hospital immediately. I went to fetch him from our home at once, and shortly after lunch we were at the hospital.

I sat beside his bed in the haematology ward. He felt awful. His body was on fire and he wheezed heavily with every breath. He could scarcely sip some fruit juice. I was taking a work call on my cellular telephone when it happened – the bed, the floor, and everything within a two metre radius of Derik, including me, was soaked by the liquid that spewed from his mouth. I cut my conversation short instantly. Derik was uncontrollably nauseous. But the nausea also brought relief, and he eventually fell into a feverish sleep.

I went home early that evening. At about eight o'clock I called the hospital to find out how he was. The sister on duty said: "Derik is currently out of danger, as his blood pressure has improved to 50 over 27." I broke into a cold sweat and started shaking as I sat on the bed in our room. "50 over 27?"

I tried to keep the receiver still. A normal blood pressure is much, much higher than that.

"Don't worry," she comforted me, "his blood pressure is better than it was earlier. At one point it was 30 over 10."

She tried to set me at ease: I could relax now. Derik had almost died, but it seemed as if everything was relatively under control. For the time being there was no reason to be concerned. They actually had wanted to call me, but Derik had not wanted them to upset me "unnecessarily" and had insisted that they not call me.

The sister gave me more details. Most fortunately, the professor had been in the vicinity when the crisis occurred. If it had not been for his immediate reaction and instructions, Derik's heart would have stopped. I did not think this was a coincidence. Apparently Derik had wanted to go to the bathroom, but was unaware that his blood pressure had dropped significantly. Because he was so weak, he stumbled into a trolley of trays. The sound of trays crashing to the ground alerted the nurses. The patients in this hall did not have individual monitors attached to them, and normally the staff would not have known how low Derik's blood pressure had dropped. It was a blessing that he had made so much noise. Nothing is accidental. It had not been Derik's time to go. I saw the incident as a sure sign that Derik would recover fully. Why else would his body have refused this golden opportunity to give in?

I was extremely distressed after the telephone call, but realised that Derik's instability could worsen if I drove to the hospital then. It was even too dangerous to speak to him on the telephone. After the experience of his temperature rising drastically on the afternoon of my iron transfusion, I had realised what a fine line there was between stability and chaos. So instead, I called Heather. I needed someone with a quiet voice and a solid presence to help me calm down. As always when she spoke to me during this time, she transferred her tranquillity to me. She has an uncanny sensitivity to the unseen world, and I eagerly held onto her vision that Derik would have a peaceful night.

—— Original Message ——
From: Momberg Marthie
Sent: Friday, 28 May 1999 10:41 AM
To: Colleagues and friends
Subject: Derik

Dear friends and colleagues
I hope you are all well.

Derik was at home for a wonderful six weeks, but yesterday he was unexpectedly taken to hospital with a fever of 41 degrees. Later in the day, his blood pressure dropped to 30 over 10 and his heart almost stopped. It is only through grace and the competent assistance of the doctor and the nursing staff that he was stabilised in time. His fever is currently under control and his blood pressure is rising slowly but steadily. We do not know what caused the fever and the drop in his blood pressure, we're still waiting for the results.

We realised once more how great the grace of God is. Both Derik and I view this incident as another opportunity to learn something about the wonder of the universe.

Thank you for your faith, your devoted energy and your prayers.
MM

The following day it was found that Derik had suffered from septic shock. During the cleaning of his J-line, some dirt must have ended up in his bloodstream. This had caused the violent reaction in his body. The incident had given everybody a huge fright, but it was over now. When I thanked the doctor for what he had done, he mentioned that Derik still had a good chance at recovery. But first, they had to get rid of the fungus in his lungs, and the doctor felt that time was running out.

Because so much time had elapsed since the last chemotherapy and because Derik had been too ill to receive the final treatment, there was a danger that the acute leukaemia could become active again and that the blast cells could return to his body. However, a fourth course of chemotherapy could weaken him so much that he would not survive a bone marrow transplant. The doctor was therefore considering moving directly to the transplant. The professor repeated that Derik still had a seventy per cent chance of recovery if he received the transplant. To our delight, two potential donors were identified in England at this time. Both still had to undergo final tests, but so far all the test results had been positive

The search for a donor had not been without incident. Normally, it takes between three and six months to find a suitable DNA structure, but more than six months had passed and a suitable donor had not yet been found. There had been some administrative carelessness at the bone marrow registry, or, as one of the hospital staff put it, the official did not think that the search was "that urgent" and so she had not responded immediately to the faxes. Thus, weeks of critical search time were lost. However, we were so grateful that Derik had survived the most recent crisis that we did not want to be upset about this. It was as if we were entering a set of rapids and simply could not control every aspect of our surroundings. Everything was moving so quickly that in some ways we simply trusted that it would work out.

Five days after Derik's blood pressure had dropped so dangerously, he was ready to come home again. But a week later, he had another fever attack and we rushed him back to the hospital. He was still weak from the previous experience, and had to be taken in a wheelchair from the car to the unit in the hospital. While we were waiting for the paperwork to be completed, I noticed the sag in his shoulders. There were black rings under his eyes and his hand clasped the irrigation pipe stand tightly. He was run down. The receptionist also noticed this, and called the unit to see whether his bed was ready yet.

"I can see that Dr Momberg is tired, he is very uncomfortable," she said over the telephone.

We were filled with a combination of anxiety and uncertainty. Both of us were tense. What was wrong this time? How many more times would something happen? When would he be ready for the final chemotherapy and the bone marrow transplant? We were greatly relieved when the two sisters who finally admitted him to the isolation ward began to tease him about being back yet again and that he apparently did not seem to enjoy being at home.

"We're getting tired of you, Derik," Savy said. "We're getting bored with your infections, you know. We only want to see you again when you come in for your transplant!"

We all laughed, and by the time Savy and Jenny had finished their monitoring and had set up the intravenous antibiotic we felt better. The strange anxiety had melted away with the laughter. The doctors would find the problem and solve it. We had to trust the process. We had received help up to now, and we would continue to do so. We would get through this too. There was no reason to be scared. We just had to trust the process. It was Thursday afternoon, 10 June.

The following evening the doctor called me at home. The professor was attending a conference abroad and a colleague was taking care of his patients. I was in bed when the telephone rang. He told me that he was very sorry to have to inform me that the blast cells were back in Derik's blood.

8

"Almost Certainly"

The blast cells were back in Derik's blood. This meant that he was no longer in remission. I do not know exactly what I felt at that moment, except that everything was now moving a bit too fast.

"What about the transplant then?" I asked. "After all, there are donors – couldn't they go ahead with the transplant?"

"No," the doctor replied. "If the blast cells are back, there is no hope of a transplant."

I sat shivering in my pyjamas. The doctor added that Derik's condition had deteriorated so much that he would probably not survive the night. His blood pressure was dropping. Even if he did survive the night, he would definitely die within the next twenty-four hours. Of this the doctor was quite sure.

I could not accept the doctor's opinion. It simply did not feel as if it was Derik's time to go. Had I not started to trust my intuition over the past few months? Of course, I could be wrong, but nothing, absolutely nothing made me feel that Derik was going to die within a day. The doctor must have heard something in the tone of my voice for he repeated firmly that I had to come to terms with the news. Was my reaction denial? I do not think so. It was more like a definite awareness that contrasted sharply with what the doctor was saying.

My whole body was shaking by the time I put the telephone down. I called the hospital immediately and asked to speak to the nurse on duty. It was no coincidence that Claire answered the telephone. She and Derik had developed a special relationship. She promised that she would stay at his bedside all night and call me immediately if she thought I should come to the hospital.

Then I called my mother. Again, it was no coincidence that my brother had arrived from Pretoria for a short visit earlier that evening. I asked them to drive to Stellenbosch and spend the night with me. Finally I called Hans and Anneke. By now my equilibrium had completely dissipated, and I could only muster sobs when Hans answered the telephone. I had probably hyperventilated as well, and could therefore not utter a sound. They were at our house within minutes.

Once they heard that Derik was not well at all, Hans left immediately for their house to start a telephone chain, asking our friends to pray for us. Anneke wrapped her arms around me, made me some tea, and we prayed together. Anneke asked the Lord to give us strength, and I asked that Derik should not suffer. We did not ask for Derik to be healed, as it did not feel right to do so to either of us. I simply knew that Derik was not about to die, but I had no idea what would happen in the future. I was numb with shock and allowed Anneke to lead me to bed and tuck the blankets in around me. Then we waited for my mother and brother to arrive – Anneke downstairs in the lounge, and me upstairs in our bed, with our cat licking the tears off my face.

The rest of the night passed without incident, and I left for the hospital at the crack of dawn. Derik was still suffering acute pain. To him it felt as if every cell in his body ached. Not even the morphine he had been given the night before could dull the pain. When he coughed, he held his chest tightly. I silently cried out for help. And then came the relief that lit up his face.

"Do you remember that lovely meal we had…?" he asked me with wonder in his eyes and a smile on his lips.

Although his blood pressure was still very low, it had stopped dropping, and he could sit up slightly to talk to me. A while later, the doctor arrived. He took a long time to examine Derik carefully and intently. He pushed down on his abdomen, listened to his heart and asked where he felt the pain. I sat on a chair on the other side of the bed. Derik watched the doctor's every move. No one spoke for almost the duration of the examination. Eventually, the doctor told Derik to take some medication to help ease the pain. I knew that what he was prescribing would provide only symptomatic relief. But it was the way in which Derik listened to him and then affirmed that he would do exactly what the doctor had suggested that remains with me. His whole being seemed to be eagerly reaching out to the doctor's words. He responded with so much gratitude that one would have thought that the doctor had offered him a miracle cure.

Then the doctor asked to speak to me and walked ahead into the hallway outside Derik's room. There he repeated that my husband would certainly not live for more than a day or two. Again I asked whether a transplant was completely out of the question. I immediately noticed the doctor's irritation. He told me emphatically that it would be better for me to come to terms with the fact that Derik was dying. I wanted to cry out "But what about God? Why can't I hope for a miracle?" As I looked into his face, I knew that that was not the thing to say at this time. So I thanked him, turned around and went back to my husband.

Of course Derik wanted to know what we had talked about. Since I did not trust the doctor's opinion, I could not tell Derik everything. This was the only time ever that I did not share the whole truth with Derik immediately. I tried to keep my voice as even and natural as possible and told him that the doctor had explained to me that his condition was very serious. Although I was outraged that the doctor had not had the courage to speak to Derik directly and was especially angry that he had asked to see me in private in front of Derik, it did mean that Derik was spared from hearing his condemning opinion. Like me, Derik remained convinced that a transplant was indeed still possible. Together we decided that it would be better to wait until the professor returned the next day and to ask him what exactly was happening.

But before the next day would dawn, we had to survive this day. I remained silently at Derik's bedside for the rest of the day while he drifted in and out of sleep. I could neither eat nor read. What if the doctor was correct? Was this indeed Derik's last day on earth? The passing of every half an hour was marked by the pumping sound of the black band around Derik's arm inflating automatically, to be followed by readings of his heart rate, oxygen levels and blood pressure by an electronic monitor. Every time I heard the pumping sound, I involuntarily drew in my breath and my own heart beat faster. And wonder above wonders, half-hour by half-hour the readings improved. Every time – decimal by decimal – there was a slight but nevertheless steady improvement.

I did not think, I was not nervous; the hysteria of the previous evening had dissipated. I had entered stormy waters and was trying to keep myself afloat. I had no control over the speed and was unable to see the hazards ahead. As his condition improved, my inner feeling that "the rapids" would eventually end somewhere and that we would once more enter calmer waters grew stronger. I just had to remain level headed.

Towards evening, Derik's blood pressure still indicated a stable improvement, and he was wide awake. I decided it was too late for me to drive home and told him that I would spend the night with my mother. I wanted to put him at ease. I also realised that I was exhausted and that I wanted to be as close to the hospital as possible. And I wanted to be nurtured. Our own home had always been a safe haven for me, but now I did not feel strong enough to return there alone. Although I did not want to believe the doctor, it would have been irresponsible to ignore his professional and very pointed opinion. It was evident that Derik was in considerable pain and it was indeed possible that he could die. How was I to know?

I had a small bowl of stewed apples for supper at my mother's home. Just as when I had told her that Derik had leukaemia, my sobs now rose from my very core. I clenched my fists and fought with untold intensity against the possibility that Derik could die. It was unacceptable to me. This was not what Derik and I wanted. Derik was not allowed to die! He simply could not die! My mother gave me a tranquillizer, then I had a bath and dressed myself in a pair of her warm woollen pyjamas. Gratefully I cuddled up in bed with a hot water bottle. Claire was still on duty, and again she assured me that she would call me immediately if I needed to come to the hospital. I was infinitely thankful that she was with Derik. Eventually, the sleeping pill took effect. During the night, I woke up and called Claire, but Derik was fine.

As soon as I woke in the morning I left for the hospital. I asked to see the professor the moment he was available. It was a Sunday, but, as always, he was there early. Ignoring the hospital regulations, I sat on Derik's bed and we talked. I told him that I had asked to see the professor so that we could find out exactly what was happening. It was shortly after eight when the sister called me – Prof J wanted to see me in the conference room just outside the unit. The professor, the senior nurse and the pharmacist were all there when I entered. I sat down on a chair, my arms on the armrests on either side, my legs uncrossed in front of me – the neutral position. He got straight to the point. My husband was very ill and there was nothing more they could do for him. If there had not been the fungal infection in his lungs, he, the doctor, could have proceeded with a transplant. However, while the infection was still present, he did not want to put Derik through another session of chemotherapy and radiation, which was what was required to destroy all the bone marrow before the transplant. The infection, compounded by the damage to his liver and kidneys and the negative effects of the chemotherapy, would be too much – Derik would not be able to survive it all.

"Your husband does not have much time left," he said. I wanted to know how much time. Then he spoke the words that have etched themselves in my memory:

"Your husband will almost certainly die within two weeks."

I could no longer remain calm. I leaned forward and covered my face with my hands. For a while, the four of us sat in silence. No words, only my sobs. Then the sister gave me some tissues. The doctor continued. There were three options: they could take care of Derik at the unit, or they could transfer him to a hospice, or he could go home and I could look after him. I responded immediately, as my choice was easy: Derik would come home with me. Very well, the doctor replied, the hospital staff would try to stabilise his blood pressure as much as possible within the next day or two so that he could go home. I thanked them and went back to Derik.

As I walked into the change room to take off the jacket that covered my pink hospital clothing, Kirsten, one of the sisters, was there. My tears started to flow uncontrollably once more and she cried with me. She held me in her arms, and I realised how heart-rending it is for the nursing staff to go through this trauma each time a patient dies.

"I **expect** a miracle," I told her.

"We will pray for you. We are all there for you," she replied.

I believed her. I knew how much they had grown to love Derik in the months he had spent in hospital and how much they wanted him to recover.

By the time I entered Derik's room I was calm. Again I sat on the bed, this time to tell him that I did not have good news. It was no longer possible to do the transplant. He listened quietly. I told him that the professor did not think he would live much longer.

"How much time have I got?" he wanted to know.

"Two weeks," I said. Derik nodded his head.

It was enough to be able to sit with each other. As always, it felt as if Derik's mere presence was enough to ease my tension. The intense anxiety of the past few days was replaced by serenity. Both of us were calm, very calm. In a strange way, we both felt relieved. We said as much to each other. The uncertainty was over and at last we knew what the road ahead held for us. In the change room I had wanted my will to prevail, but now I accepted the message. We spent the rest of the day together quietly. Derik slept for most of the time, and I read Gideon Joubert's *Die Groot Gedagte* (The Great Thought). It was a good day.

Later, I went back to my mother's home in Welgemoed. This time, she gave me a sleeping pill as soon as I entered the house, and I accepted it gratefully. For the first time in two days I was able to eat something more substantial – an egg on toast and a cup of tea.

But in my room, lying alone on my bed, raw emotion overcame me. Peace and acceptance disappeared and the uncertainty returned. I was in so much emotional pain that I felt as if I wanted to tear the clothes off my body. If I had been able, I would have torn off my skin as well. It was a strong, penetrating physical pain – my heart literally ached. I held my head in my hands and entered into a deep discussion with God.

I explained to Him the sharp division in my thoughts. On the one hand, the specialists were clearly convinced that Derik was dying. On the other, nothing inside me felt that this was true. I did not know what to believe or think. I did not want stubbornly to continue believing that Derik would live if this was not meant to be. But I also did not want to accept that he was dying simply because the specialists had said so. How was I to know what God's will was? If He intended Derik to die right now, I was willing to accept it, **but** He had to give me this message Himself. The doctors based their opinions on their knowledge and experience of similar situations, but this only encompasses a tiny portion of reality. I had already begun to discover that reality did not comprise only the visible and therefore I could not accept their word as the complete reality.

It was also important to know whether Derik still **wanted** to live. If he felt that he had reached the end of his earthly existence, I could accept his death. I had to gain clarity about God's will, and about Derik's will, before I would accept anything. Under no circumstances did I want my personal desires to count at Derik's expense. This was not about my life in the first place, and I had no right to demand Derik's health. What I did expect, however, was to know what to think about the future. Therefore I asked God to give me a clear signal – I wanted to know whether I dared to hope or if I should accept the medical opinion. Whatever the answer, I would acquiesce.

Once again Claire sat at Derik's bedside that night, and once again I got up as early as possible to go to the hospital. It was Monday, 14 June. Just before I left, I asked my mother to contact a friend, Sandra, in Stellenbosch. Sandra was the chairperson of the Hospice Association in the Western Cape, and I realised that I would need their help at home. It was not yet eight o'clock when I walked into Derik's room, but he already had a visitor – Piet du Plooy from Windhoek.

Piet and his wife Ilsje had called me from Namibia some months earlier. I had not known them at all, but we did have mutual friends in Stellenbosch. Piet was a former Matie rugby captain and a top sportsman who had contracted acute myeloid leukaemia a few years before. He had also been treated by Prof J and had turned at death's door before recovering fully. During the months of Derik's illness, Piet and Ilsje called me almost every week to lend their support. They came to visit us every time they came to Cape Town. Now Piet was here beside Derik, solid and strong.

As I walked into the room he put his hands around Derik's aching feet with these words, "Remember, never stop hoping."

My first thought was "Are you crazy? How can you say that to Derik? Don't you know what the doctor said?"

Piet was well aware of what the doctor had said, but he knew from his own experience that miracles do happen. While I stood there looking at Piet, the significance of his words penetrated. Hope – was this not the answer I was seeking?

"Remember, never, ever give up hope," he repeated and put his hands firmly around Derik's feet.

When Piet left I walked out with him to say goodbye. As he held me to him, I felt some of his strength seeping into me.

On my return, Derik was sitting up in bed. He still cringed with pain whenever he coughed; yet he was looking markedly better. There was a brightness about his face when he said: "I have decided to hope again."

"So have I," I heard myself answer. I had asked for a sign, and here I had walked into my husband's room early in the morning and the first words I heard were "Don't ever stop hoping."

Once more, my fears and anxieties were washed away by Derik's presence. The mere fact that he was there made me feel safe and protected. It was as if my deepest being was untouchable even by death when I was with him.

Derik put deed to word. For the past while I had had to help him whenever he had needed to go to the bathroom. Today, however, he was going to get out of bed because if he wanted to go home, he would have to help himself.

A while later, I walked into Savy, the head nurse, in the corridor. She had just arrived at work after having had the weekend off. When I had last seen her on Friday, she had made us laugh when she had joked about Derik's incessant infections. Now she came over to me, repeating over and over again, "I'm so sorry, oh Marthie. I didn't know… I'm so sorry." I was unable to answer and started to cry. Gently she led me to the nurses' lounge, and what she then did had a profound effect on my life.

In her quiet tone Savy started speaking to me. "Let me tell you something…" she said.

She told me that years of working in the transplant unit had taught her one thing – one should never give up hope. Savy had already seen many patients die, but what she chose to share with me was that I should never give up hope. I was astounded. I had expected her to give me the medical facts, but that was not what she did.

She proceeded to point out that she had twice seen the impossible become a reality. One of these was her experience with Piet du Plooy. While she was talking to me, one of the other sisters peeked in, but closed the door behind her without interrupting us. Savy took my hands in hers and prayed for me in a way that no one had ever prayed for me before. I was moved by the power of her emotion, and she showed me how one can beg for mercy from God when one is feeling helpless. Once more, the door of the lounge opened and closed. Savy was still talking to me when the door opened for a third time.

"Marthie," the nurse at the door said, "Derik wants you to come to him."

I must have spent a long time with Savy – I have no idea how long – but when I walked out of the lounge to go to Derik, I felt as if I was much, much bigger than my body. It was as if my innermost self had finally burst forth and had enveloped me in a totally new, all-inclusive and intense joyous energy.

Derik was convulsed with fever. "Where were you?" he demanded shakily.

I quickly explained and apologised for leaving him on his own for so long. After two fever-free days, Derik's temperature had suddenly risen to almost 41 degrees. Coupled with the still low blood pressure, this could be deadly, but not even this could touch me now. I was light, light and free; detached from fear. I felt elated.

My mother and brother stood at the end of the bed, shocked. They had popped in briefly to see Derik and were confronted with a convulsing, shivering being. They did not know what to do. I covered Derik with more bedding and pulled on his woollen cap. Nothing helped. It was a massive fever attack that flung his weakened body back and forth. I tried to set my mother and brother at ease and pressed the button to call the nurse – perhaps she could give him a suppository to combat the horrific fever.

I had no doubt whatsoever that the fever would break. In the meantime, I tried to regulate Derik's breathing. With my head near his, we breathed together – in, out, in, out, I instructed him. We remained like this for some time – my brother and mother standing tensely at the end of the bed, and me at his head. Where was the sister? Why was no one coming to help us?

Derik broke the rhythm: "My dear, please, your breath smells awful. Can't you please move your head?"

Derik transferred us immediately from the portals of death into the present. My mother, my brother and I burst out laughing. It had been three days since I had been at home, and I had been coping with only the bare essentials. My breath must indeed have been really foul as for three days I had only rinsed my mouth. We were clinging to the bed screaming with laughter when the nurse walked in. It must have been a very odd sight.

Despite the relief the laughter had brought, my mother and brother were utterly confused and distressed. They felt that they would not see Derik again. When they left I reassured them that they need not worry – Derik would get better and he was not going to die right away. I was truly liberated from any fear. However, they were so flustered and disoriented that they struggled to find their way out of the unit and the twenty-minute journey home took them two hours.

I stayed with Derik until the fever broke, and in this time had one of the most incredible and uplifting experiences of my life. Any fear of death in me dissipated. I was set free. Death could not touch me. While I was standing next to him, I told the invisible presences in the room that they could leave; they were in the wrong place at the wrong time. There was an enormous energy in me that filled the whole room. It felt as if the force within and surrounding me had done an about turn. It was not a mere emotion or a figment of my imagination, it was a genuine sensation – something like a strong wind that whirled through me and the glowing atmosphere around me. I was deeply aware of this concrete change in my energy. It was as if my heart, my mind and my soul brightened, as if they were filled with Light, as if I was one with God and the world. An unutterable love, joy and certainty enveloped me. It was almost too much to contain. Like a protector, I watched over Derik, who now seemed to be unaware of his surroundings. Nothing, absolutely nothing would happen to him against his will.

I ordered myself some lunch and devoured it hungrily as I sat beside my sleeping husband.

It was impossible for the people around us to understand what was happening to us or to know what we thought. I had no words to describe it. My mother and my brother could not comprehend how I managed to appear in such high spirits and why I kept telling them that Derik was not dying. The shock of the morning's experience was still with them. Like many of our friends at a later stage, they were concerned that I was denying the reality. Some people thought that I felt responsible for Derik's life – that if he died, I would feel as if I had failed. Derik's mother and his sister did not believe that Derik would live for more than two weeks and insisted on saying their goodbyes.

I had wanted with my whole heart to be with Derik for many more years, and now I had the certainty that he had not yet reached the end of his life. I only began to understand my new-found energy much later, but at that stage, my greatest breakthrough was that I could look at Derik as someone who was **alive** and not as someone who was dying. I therefore defined our existence in terms of light and life, and not in terms of departure and death.

Our godchild, Carin, had told me after she had lived through her mother's illness and death that if one stops hoping, one stops living. Now I understood her. For the first time I could also understand why our friends Christo and Liesel Greyling called their anti-AIDS campaign "I have hope". If we had walked out of the hospital with death, we would have stopped living that morning. However, we both chose to walk out of there with hope – so that we would continue to live for every day that followed. That was the most important thing.

As had become the custom, my mother was ready with a tranquilliser and sleeping pill when I arrived at her home.

I refused them. I knew that I no longer needed these pills. It had been a very good day. I had asked for a sign and received three very clear signs through Piet, Derik and Savy. I also held onto what Prof J had said: "Your husband will almost certainly die very soon." **Almost certainly**, I kept telling myself, **almost certainly**. By saying this, the doctor had admitted that he was not God. He had done everything in his power to help Derik. On the grounds of his own previous experience, he could predict that Derik would die within two weeks, but he could not guarantee this.

By Tuesday morning, the remarkable change in Derik was clearly noticeable. He could go to the bathroom by himself, and he dressed himself in his new bottle-green tracksuit. I packed the rest of his belongings and then we were ready for his discharge. I called my mother to tell her that she could let Sandra know that we no longer needed the Hospice's assistance.

The rays of the winter sun stretched across Derik's bed while the sister explained which medicines he could use at home. There were various painkillers, medication to help clot his blood, something to keep his blood thin, something for nausea and diarrhoea, different types of antibiotics, vitamins, minerals and liquid meals. Bags full of pills and a page full of instructions, none of which contained a cure for leukaemia. The professor came to say goodbye. It was obvious that he found it very difficult. As far as possible, he tried to comfort us. "Two, maybe three weeks," he told Derik.

Wouter was lying in the room opposite Derik, but I did not have the courage to say goodbye to him. He should have had his transplant weeks ago, but had also contracted a serious infection in his lungs. If he knew that Derik had been finally discharged, it would have broken his spirit. The sister who had looked after Derik during his last few days in hospital hugged us and assured us that she would ceaselessly pray for us. We were grateful that the other staff members were all busy elsewhere and did not see us walking down the hallway. Derik was too weak to walk by himself, and I pushed him in a wheelchair – out through the double doors that separated the unit from the rest of the building, down the hospital passage to our car, which was parked right in front of the main entrance. There was a sense of triumph as we walked out of the hospital. We knew that Derik would never return, that this phase had passed by for ever. And it was good. As I pushed Derik down the passage, he said to me, "Now I'm flying solo."

Two months later, with spring already approaching, Derik reflected on his stay in hospital and his homecoming as follows:

my darling wife

> your warm back basks against me deep at night when all
> has grown quiet around us
> you lean against me like the brown woollen karos on our
>   bed
> and together we dream dreams of who-knows-where and
>   who-knows-when
> of foreign warm white beaches with clear blue waters
> to unknown cities and mountains that lie yet unconquered
> and strange lands and cultures where we can still learn
> together we drink a toast
> to health and to love
> until our longings wake in the watch of dawn
> once more aware of each other's earthly presence
> in isolation, this was taken from me, seized
> and as a substitute I was offered a room at 21 degrees

the substitute conditioning was almost perfected
your first touch strange, intrusive
my skin no longer knew the warmth of another

but you were my strength, my second
without expectation, without conditions
you were there when I needed you
you led me when I no longer could
you sponged me when my hand could no longer hold
and taught me to walk when I could no longer crawl
you were there when I crossed the finishing line in a
 wheelchair

your laughter like a molecule is bound to the smell of
 narcissus that surrounds you
the fragrance of freesias, wisteria and jasmine mingles with
 your being
there for me to discover anew, to experience in my child-
 hood
your storytelling left child and adult awestruck:
gnomes and fairies that travel to your trees on moonlit
 evenings
painting your flower forest in rainbow colours
that which the unbeliever or nihilist could not discover even
 by day
or the sense of humour with which God created you
you coloured the shades of our lives
your fine hands shaped the potter's clay directing our
 existence
so that I could enter the fourth dimension
where sound and music mingle with angel choirs
without the cacophony of man-made mammon
you are my darling girl, you are my dearest wife

you are my summer and winter
you are my autumn and spring
you are my closest friend because water is wet
you are mine, heart-spinning lady thief
I could eat you all up

9

Completing the First Cycle

In the hospital, Derik and I had agreed to invite a group of friends over the day after his discharge. We realised that we could not travel this road alone – we needed their help. Theunis, our minister, was there, as well as Bart and Marjanne who would arrange meals, Hans and Anneke who would be in charge of our telephone information chain and Johann, Tienie and Anneliese, our medical friends.

> Dear Derik and Marthie
> How can I ever forget 16 June 1999? It is the last 16 June of the century; it is Youth Day, on which we commemorate the tragedy of 16 June 1976; our new State President is being inaugurated today; on the cricket pitch, two teams are fighting for a place in the finals of the World Cup – the winner will face either South Africa or Australia, and in KwaZulu-Natal, thousands of people are running the gruelling Comrades Marathon. But in Stellenbosch, a tiny group of people are gathered in Cynaroides Street, Paradyskloof, in the champagne light of a winter's day – all of them commandeered to be there by you.
> At a first glimpse, what we all have in common is the special place the two of you hold in our hearts. The gathering starts off subdued and tense. Each of us has an inkling of what the agenda will be. You are quiet at this stage, Derik,

and Marthie is busy somewhere in the house. But then, out come the aromatic coffee, tea and something sweet and we bring more chairs out onto the veranda and spontaneously encircle you. You break the ice and lead us into the world of your emotions and thoughts. You cry and try to overcome the lump in your throat, and yet, without your having to explain, we know: life is precious, friends are precious, and the thought of losing either touch us deeply. Tears flow freely from our eyes as well.

You display more control as you share what's going on – your hospitalisation last week, the doctor's verdict. The destructive effects of the antibiotics, the damage to your kidneys and liver, and the return of the cancer cells... We listen intently and then you cast the net around us – you need us. Suddenly, we are no longer just a group of individuals to whom you are special, we become a team, a core team to whom you would like to come without reservation when and wherever necessary.

You give thanks to your Maker, in whose hands you have placed yourself and you soberly invite us to accompany you down the road you are about to travel. You don't know where it leads, but you are going to walk down it. We nod, we agree, we express our solidarity... we want to go... we do!

And Marthie, you help us to perceive both of you in new ways... with our consciousness... to look with God, the God who heals. You radiate peace, because the worst is over. Derik is alive. You are ready to release. You are in God's hands, and you will continue to live your lives from there. You have hope.

I do too! Thank you for making me a part of your lives, and also that I can be part of God's healing process.

We have some more coffee and you show all the medicines to the doctors in our presence. We form a circle once more before we continue with the rest of the day, pillared against the Rock who is our resting place and our salvation (Ps 62).

I drive home with a happy heart! I commit you both to God again, and again, and again.

Theunis B.

I took three weeks' leave. But I did not want to spend this time preparing meals and doing other chores; I rather wanted to be wholly with Derik all the time. One of the requests to our support team was therefore that they help to prepare a cooked meal that conformed to the hospital's specifications every day. Derik's immunity was still very low, and we wanted to stick to the dietary guidelines. Furthermore, the food had to be soft enough for Derik to eat. I thought I was asking our friends a huge favour, but their response was so overwhelming that it felt as if we were in fact doing them a favour. Night after night our doorbell rang at seven o'clock and, when I opened the door, there stood someone holding a tray with a freshly cooked hot meal.

On the first night, Marjanne made us Dutch pea soup. Bart brought the food over and made a fire in our hearth. Derik had left the hospital in a wheelchair that morning, had survived the journey from Plumstead to Stellenbosch and had walked from the car to the house on his own. These were massive achievements for someone who was so sick and weak that the doctors felt he was going to die soon. He was lying on the couch in the lounge, his grossly swollen feet resting on cushions, when Bart brought the soup in. Derik revelled in the warmth of the fire and the aroma of the soup, but could manage to eat only a few spoonfuls with my assistance. I could sense Bart's dismay. What Derik and I saw as significant improvements, looked like tremendous deterioration – the behaviour of a very, very sick person – to Bart. Yet the three of us were merely seeing different aspects of the same reality. There were probably more aspects of which we were not even aware. None of us knew what the complete reality was. Everything is relative, and it all depends on the perspective from which one views a matter.

Derik fell into a deep sleep on his couch, while Bart and I sat on the other couch and ate our supper. That evening I realised how radically Derik's process was affecting our friends. Bart cried like a baby over his friend with whom he had gone hiking, swimming and diving, and he spoke about how he was trying to make sense of circumstances such as ours. He knew Derik as someone who was always resourceful. "MacGyver" he called him, because Derik could fashion a shelter from virtually nothing in the veld; he could perform tricks with his penknife, to great delight, for he invariably cut his finger at the climax of each of his "performances". And he had inspired Bart, the engineer, to become the owner-builder of his own house. It was not only me, Derik and our family who were touched by his illness: many of the people around us were also affected. Derik's illness had given us all the opportunity to reflect.

In our search for the meaning of life, the point of departure is often a search for our own purpose in life. We try to establish how we have to grow and develop. If something untoward or extraordinary happens to us, we think that it happens because the "self" needs to grow. But how do we define this "self"? Who are we? Is it the individual? Is it all of us collectively? Can something happen to one person without its affecting others? I do not think so. When it concerns the "self", it also concerns the people around this "self". I accept that we are of the same Body, that we are part of God and that we are therefore part of one another. We are One. Whatever happens to us, affects those who surround us, it "happens" to them as well.

That which we experience fits into a larger plan of which we are not always aware. "Our knowledge and our prophecy alike are partial" (1 Cor. 13:9). We perceive only aspects of reality, and often we are blind to the connections between events. I believe that this plan was created by God, but that it works in a way that allows us to be more than mere victims of predestination. That is why we have a will, emotions and a mind, and why we can choose how we are going to respond to specific circumstances. If we believe that God is in control of this plan and that we are part of God, then we can also deduce that whatever happens to us is not just God's doing, but also our own.

Is it therefore possible that something can deliberately happen to one person so that it can also bring about change in another? Derik and I decided that it could indeed be so. It was obvious to us that our processes and experiences had found resonance in the lives and experiences of our friends, colleagues and families. Actually, it goes even deeper. Our own experiences of love, life, death, hope, fear and trust are complemented and shaped by the experiences of our loved ones. Like a mosaic that is formed over time by adding many little pieces, each with its own colour, shape and size, our own experience was taking shape through the vision, the dreams, the hope and despair, and the closeness or distancing of those around us. There was a relationship between who and what we were and the world around us. Some parts were necessary to form the background, while others formed an integral part of the picture itself. To leave out even one piece of the mosaic, would mean that the picture could not be completed. No one could therefore have a less important role than anyone else. Every person had a unique function. One person's hope sustained us in a particular way, just as another's despair did. It was precisely the fears of some that helped us to understand what we ourselves believed, and the distancing of others that made us realise that the emotion of our process was too much for them to manage within the allotted time. We were not the only brittle beings. Derik and I felt greatly privileged to be given the opportunity to walk this path of life or death consciously.

We did not know for how long Derik would live, but took comfort in the fact that the rest of the process would not only be to our advantage, but would benefit those around us as well. If he was going to die, Derik told me, he wanted his death to mean something to others as well.

Our conception of "life" and "death" also began to alter, along with the last grain of fear. Up to now we had thought it necessary for Derik to recover completely. But what constituted "health"? We began to realise that "health" did not necessarily include complete physical healing. Life and death now became relative concepts. Death was not an end; birth was not a beginning. Rather, the one was a continuation of the other, in a different dimension. Why, therefore, would a person attempt to stay on earth with all the power of this world if he was destined to enter a wonderful new dimension? Do Christians not believe that a wonderful life lies at the end of our earthly life, and that life on earth is not the final goal?

It is human not to want to take leave of one's loved ones or of what one knows. It is like standing on a tall rock and being afraid to jump into the water below. On the rock a person feels safe and sees no reason to take the plunge. But when that person eventually does jump, he discovers an immense freedom and realises that whatever he feared is actually much more rewarding and very different from what he had imagined. If we are not prepared to take the plunge, it is because our own fears prevent us from doing so.

Finally, our definition of "perfection" also changed. We no longer thought that it meant that everything had to be "perfect" – good health, secure finances, a good job, a happy marriage, beautiful children, and being talented. We realised that none of these could bring perfection. True perfection lay in the ability to find sense and happiness in the here and now, within oneself, irrespective of the circumstances.

It was these concepts, the definitions of "life", "death" and "perfection", that we mulled over during the weeks after Derik's discharge. We had a unique opportunity to tackle every day, every minute, in full consciousness.

None of these insights changed our desire for a miracle. Both of us still vehemently hoped and believed that Derik would yet recover fully. We loved each other and we wanted to continue to enjoy life together. We had ideals and plans for the future. Sometimes when people are told by respected doctors that they are going to die, they accept this as a reality and prepare themselves accordingly. We did not do this, because it did not **feel** right in our particular circumstances. We did not deny the possibility that Derik could die within a couple of weeks; we just knew that this was not going to happen.

So, on the one hand, we had new insights into life and death and, on the other, we held an intense hope for a miracle – an unshakeable trust in the unseen. We could surrender life, yet we also hoped for it. We accepted death as a wonderful new dimension, but we did not want it to enter our lives right away. We were living with two views that were diametrically opposed to each other.

Yet there was a subtle difference. In the past, we **needed** his body to heal completely. Now we no longer saw this as a necessity, but it remained our **choice**.

We lived our hope to the full. Every day constituted a lifetime, and every instant within it was precious. Every action was a step ahead in the direction of strength and health. Every second hour, when we took Derik's temperature and found it to be normal, was a step away from infection. Every gram he gained indicated an improvement. Our hope grew as the swelling in his feet subsided and the intense pain in his chest diminished. From being barely able to eat on the night of his discharge, and falling asleep on the couch, Derik advanced to where he could put on shoes, sit and walk by himself, eat small but complete meals and meditate with me in the evenings in our leather chairs in front of the hearth.

Just four days after Derik was discharged (although it felt like an eternity to us), we went for breakfast in town on the Saturday morning. We woke up early and saw that it was a crystal clear winter's day. We had already considered doing this the night before – for years it had been our custom to go to town on Saturday mornings for breakfast or for coffee, and it would be nice to do so again. Once we saw that it was a truly beautiful morning, everything seemed to point towards our going out. So we got up and, while it was still quiet outside, drove to town. On our way we realised that we were heading for the same place at which we had had our last meal together before Derik was hospitalised seven months before. We were completing a circle.

The significance of this morning lay not only in the fact that we (coincidentally?) were en route to the same place, but that it was also the first time that we were publicly enjoying an entire "outing" together. The breakfast became a symbol of a new beginning. We had thought that our last meal at De Ouwe Werf would mark the end of our lives together, that we were taking leave and that Derik would never come home again. How wrong we had been. It had merely been the start of the hospital phase, and now we stood once more at the beginning of a new phase.

For the first time in months, we were able to perform a "normal" activity. It was only a week since I had anxiously watched over Derik while his blood pressure rose decimal by decimal. Now no one was looking at us. We could walk into a restaurant as if by chance, unnoticed, as if it was the most ordinary thing in the world to do, ask for a table for two and be seated. The waitress greeted us like any other couple who wanted to have bacon and eggs. Of course, she was extremely professional in her service, but we realised from her expression that she did not see anything extraordinary about us. We ordered our food and realised that no one in the restaurant was looking at us. We were perfectly normal. On that sunny day in June, a scrawny man with short hair and a woman with curly hair of medium length sat at a table with a white tablecloth and fresh flowers and ate an English breakfast. It was as if nothing had ever happened to them. That was 19 June, exactly four months before 19 October 1999.

Our loved ones heeded the doctor's words and, although they did not say so directly, they all wanted to come to say their farewells in the weeks after Derik's discharge. They came alone as well as in groups, according to a strict schedule that did not allow for unexpected visitors. Without exception each one was surprised to see a person who literally radiated life. They started to remark that a miracle was happening before their eyes. Instead of getting weaker, Derik was getting stronger. When he received visitors, Derik spoke about their interests. Whenever friends and colleagues left, they expressed their amazement at his vitality, the sharpness of his brain and his warm enthusiasm in daily events. I silently thought that at last everything was going according to plan – Derik was not dying.

Small tasks like getting up in the morning, washing and dressing still took a considerable amount of time. This was not only because Derik was still very weak, but also because we deliberately set a casual pace so that we could spend time together. Derik was not taking part in a sprint. His symbolic steps were short and small, but regular and persistent, like those of a long-distance athlete in a marathon. He had a long-term vision. As the days passed without complications, his tread grew stronger. The blood pressure monitor that Johann had left in the room remained untouched. We went to town more often – for coffee, for lunch, for tea and cake, to see a movie. It was as if we were trying to make up for lost time. We were able to walk down the street again under the bare oaks, past the whitewashed buildings. I could hook my arm into Derik's once more and walk contentedly beside my husband.

One evening after we had meditated and Derik had done his visualisation, he told me that for the first time he had had a distinct awareness that he was going to be healed completely. From a medical perspective, a cure was out of the question, but to us, who were becoming more aware of the unseen reality, nothing was impossible. To us the apparent stumbling blocks were of no concern.

In the third week after his discharge, we went back to the hospital for a follow-up visit to the stomatologist because the antiseptic cord was still in the cavity in Derik's cheek. The hollow that was filled with cord would need attention sooner or later. Derik also wanted to have his blood tested so that he could find out what was happening to his leukocyte count. It was a visit that aroused mixed emotions.

The surgeon was genuinely surprised to see how well Derik looked. He did not know that Derik was supposed to be dying, so he did not view or approach him from that perspective. Even after we had informed him of the state of affairs, he treated Derik as someone who had a right to life.

By contrast, the visit to the haematology clinic came as an unexpected and chilling experience. The administrative staff were very professional in the way they treated us, but for the first time we noticed a distance. Derik was no longer a patient who could be helped and could therefore no longer be welcomed there. He was "on the other side", so to speak. He was not expected to live, but rather to die soon. I was shocked that people could react in that way despite Derik's visible sense of well-being. While Derik was lying in the day ward waiting to have his blood drawn, our doctor's colleague walked in. The man who had told me to make peace with the fact that Derik was dying now avoided making eye contact with us. It was as if we did not exist. We greeted him, but he turned his back on us and spoke to the patient beside Derik. When we thought about it later, we could not blame him. It cannot be easy to be constantly facing death with someone. Nor can a doctor become emotionally involved with every patient – this would undoubtedly affect his work negatively. But at the time, it was like a dash of cold water in our faces. Thankfully, the sister who came to give us the results of the blood tests was warm and sympathetic and genuinely happy for us that the leukocyte count looked so good (it was 12, thus within the normal range). From where we stood talking to Savy through the security gates of the bone marrow transplant unit, we could see that she, too, was excited by the fact that Derik looked so well and that he had colour under his nails once more.

As we walked out past the hospital restaurant, my eyes met those of the doctor who apparently had not wanted to greet us earlier. He was having a meal with two other staff members. Immediately he looked down at his food, as if he had not seen us. We had therefore not imagined that he had avoided us in the ward. The other two staff members also allowed us to pass by "unnoticed". I do not know whether Derik saw them or not. I pulled my shoulders back slightly and walked past them with Derik at my side. It was clear that they were avoiding contact with us, but, I told myself, we had no reason whatsoever to feel guilty, ashamed or uncomfortable in any way.

―― Original Message ――
From: Momberg Marthie
Sent: Monday, 5 July 1999 2:17 PM
To: Colleagues
Subject: Good news

Dear friends and colleagues
It's truly a pleasure to write to you all today.

Roughly seven months ago, when Derik was first hospitalised, I literally sat with my hands in my hair. I was at my wits end and felt helpless. Then I realised that I could ask for help. So I wrote my first e-mail to you and I phoned all our family and friends. I asked for your prayers, your positive energy, your thoughts. And you responded overwhelmingly. You carried us for the seven months that followed.

Then, three weeks ago, we were told that Derik would live no longer than another two or three weeks. During this time, you again supported us with your energy and your prayers. No wonder Derik felt better each day. Three weeks ago he was unable to walk and eat. Yesterday, we walked three kilometres and today he returned to work (part-time to start with).

We know that God is revealing Himself through the wonderful recovery he is facilitating in Derik. We thank Him for the health Derik enjoys every day.

How can I ever thank you for your love and support?
MM

At the end of each day, when I counted out Derik's pills, I thought that another day had passed and that we were yet another day closer to proving that he did not have only two or three weeks to live. When this "waiting period" was over, Derik decided to return to work. We certainly experienced this as a miracle. He was still alive, he was not wasting away, he wanted to work again!

10

The Turning Point

The joy of his colleagues was enormous. One of them wrote to me:

"It's wonderful to see Derik here today. We had quite a party in his office this morning and he thoroughly enjoyed all the attention (mostly from the ladies it seems…)"

Derik felt good to be back. He was certainly not optimally productive, but his colleagues allowed him to become part of normal life once more. He went to the office with me three times a week, and worked at home for the rest of the time. His work had become a haven to him, a sign of life and progress. On the days he went to the office, we met for lunch together at the restaurant in the building – a daily break we both desperately needed.

I also enjoyed being back at work, as I had just heard that my team members and I had retained our positions in the newly restructured division. This announcement had been preceded by months of uncertainty about our future and the loss of many positions within the company.

Although we appeared to be functioning normally and although our daily routine comprised everyday activities, Derik and I remained intensely aware of the unusualness of the situation. He was supposed to be dying, or at least withering away, but he was attending meetings, developing market strategies and delivering presentations.

His leukocyte counts had already started rising in his first three weeks at home – proof that the leukaemia was indeed active in his body. Physically he looked and felt so well that it was hard to believe that he was suffering from an incurable terminal illness. Neither of our house doctors could accept that there was nothing that could be done for Derik. Why was he not dead, as everyone had predicted? How was it possible that daily he was growing stronger with increased vitality? No one could have believed that a man who only a few weeks before had been doubled up with pain, with barely any blood pressure and who had been unable to eat or walk was now able to drive his own car and work again!

Both our doctor friends telephoned the professor independently to ask whether Derik could not have a transplant after all. As Derik and I suspected, the professor stuck to his views. He knew that Derik looked and felt well because there were enough white blood cells in his body, but if he was to undergo another round of chemotherapy and radiation in preparation for a transplant, the infection in his lungs would gain the upper hand. We were therefore not disappointed or shocked when the professor reaffirmed his view to the general practitioners. Now they had to face up to the final facts, just as we had had to do a few weeks earlier.

Our hope for Derik's survival was not grounded in what the medical profession could do for him. That Derik and I continued to hope despite the lack of a medical solution was difficult for some people to comprehend. Others were sceptical of our hope and felt that we were being unrealistic and that we should rather be taking leave of each other and making our peace with death. This reaction was to be expected, and we understood it completely. Our behaviour may have appeared to be denial. We did not try to justify our actions – we did not want to spend any energy on that.

Derik's leukocyte counts continued to rise, but he also kept feeling better. When the professor heard how well he was doing in spite of the rising white blood count, he prescribed medication that would temporarily suppress his bone marrow. We knew from the outset that this would treat only the symptoms and that at some point his body would no longer react to the treatment.

The medication immediately had the desired effect and his leukocyte counts dropped drastically and constantly. Johann, Derik's running and flying partner and our family doctor, confirmed the positive effect of the medication on a sunny Saturday morning on the runway of the Stellenbosch airfield, right after he had received the results of the latest blood tests. We could not have received better news before spending an hour flying over False Bay with Johann. The sky was a bright, windless blue as we soared past the Strand, along to Muizenberg, around Cape Point, over Hout Bay and Kommetjie to Robben Island and then back to the mainland.

Derik felt wonderfully energetic and his symptoms were under control. To stop his counts from dropping too far and thus lowering his resistance to infection, he had to reduce the number of capsules he was taking in time. The turning point came during a weekend in Hermanus with Tjuks and Susan. It was as if we had completed another circle. These were the same friends we had visited sixteen months earlier in Hangklip the night before Derik was diagnosed with leukaemia. Now we were together again for a weekend at the sea – our first and last weekend away after his discharge from the hospital.

It was August, the season in which whales migrate from the cold Antarctic to calve in the warmer Cape waters. Our friends had rented a house right by the sea and invited us to spend a long weekend there with them. The sea thundered outside in the dark where Derik had parked our car, but inside the house there was light. A fire burned in the hearth, and Tjuks grilled some fish on it. Our room was cosy and warm.

That evening, as we crawled under the down duvet, Derik said that he was going to start reducing the medication that kept his leukocyte count under control so that it did not drop too far. He based his decision on the most recent blood test results we had received earlier in the day. The necessity to do this was confirmed by our doctor a few days later.

I will always remember that weekend as an opportunity for a most welcome rest. Tjuks and Susan spoilt us thoroughly. I relaxed while Tjuks massaged my feet; I soaked in a bath filled with aromatic bubbles that my dear friend had run for me; and I did not have to feel guilty about curling up to sleep in the middle of the day. Susan and I went for long walks while Tjuks caught fish and Derik buried himself in a book. Every meal was a high point with scrumptious food that we all enjoyed, particularly Derik. His appetite knew no bounds and it was wonderful to see him tuck in with great relish. In the bay in front of the house, the whales lifted their tails out of the water and gambolled with their newborn calves. We left with two sheaves of fynbos, warm hearts and the details of a guesthouse at which we were planning to spend a future weekend.

— Original Message —
From: Momberg Marthie
Sent: Wednesday, 18 August 1999 11:45 AM
To: Colleagues
Subject: Derik

Dear friends
It is now two months since Derik came home. Since then, he has made steady progress. Although his blood profile has

fluctuated, he has gained weight, has more energy and his lung infection is also much better. There is no possibility of a transplant, so Derik cannot be healed through any conventional medical procedures or treatments.

Yet our day-to-day living is very close to normal. Therefore we stay positive and thank God for each day's miracles.

Enjoy your work!

MM

Sometime in August, Derik at last agreed to visit the physician who offered complementary treatment. He knew that I had respected his earlier decision not to see this physician, but I had mentioned again that I wanted him to go, although I did emphasise that he had to make the decision himself. The matter rested until one Sunday evening, on the television programme *Carte Blanche*, we saw how a veterinarian had saved the lives of horses suffering from deadly equine disease by using homeopathic medicine. At the end of the programme, Derik said that he wanted to go to the doctor in Paarl.

The doctor identified the specific fungus in Derik's lungs. He gave him a herbal remedy and predicted that the fungus would disappear within a month. Derik agreed to take these capsules in addition to the supplements and medication he was already taking, for it was this fungus that prevented the professor from proceeding with a bone marrow transplant. A month later, the fungus was gone, but it was too late. Shortly after Derik had started decreasing the medication in Hermanus, it became apparent that it was no longer keeping his leukocytes under control – not even when the dosage was increased again. His bone marrow started producing immature white blood cells at an alarming rate, and also made too few red blood cells and platelets. Regular blood transfusions helped him feel better for a few days, but then the fatigue returned.

Although the fungus had been destroyed, the leukaemia was now so acute that a transplant was out of the question.

Early in September, Derik and his manager decided that he should stop working and ask to be declared unfit for work. This decision could be reviewed every six months for a fixed period so that the employee could have the opportunity of returning to work if his or her condition improved. We both accepted the decision with relief. Derik was too tired to travel from Stellenbosch to Cape Town every day. His strength was diminishing daily. Our lives were now taking a different course. On our way home after his last day at work Derik told me that he would not return to the building in Pinelands.

"When I walked out of there today, I knew that I would never return. I just know it," he remarked quietly.

He finally wanted to start writing his book. Although it was obvious that the leukaemia was very active, we both remained hopeful of a future together. Almost three months and the experiences of a lifetime had passed since we had heard in June that he was going to die. We would continue to live every day. Eighteen months ago when we had sat crying on the steps in our home, Derik had decided to resign in the near future so that he could devote his time to writing a book. In this book he wanted to integrate his thinking, his experiences in theology, psychology and the business world with his ability to observe tendencies in a fictional narrative.

The fact that he had now been declared unfit for work offered him an opportunity to make his dream come true. Nevertheless, I cried at dinner that Friday evening when Derik told our friends Attie and Carina that he was not going to work any more.

It was September, the month of Derik's birthday and also the month in which we planned to have a thanksgiving ceremony for our friends.

I went to my office in Pinelands daily, but occasionally I worked from home. Every morning before I left, Derik would ask me not to come home too late.

Derik's mother had once again travelled from Pretoria to help us. It was a visit we all enjoyed thoroughly. We also wanted her to attend the thanksgiving service for our friends and colleagues. We had decided months before to thank our loved ones for their wonderful support and felt that now was the time to do so. One of our friends, Anette C, helped us to plan a simple occasion with candles, arum lilies and a dinner.

At the beginning of September, Derik's eyesight started to deteriorate. I took him to an ophthalmologist who, to our relief, told us that the damage was reversible. Wonder above wonders, it was only fluid in his eyes, and not bleeding as is often the case with people who suffer from leukaemia. We had to wait for two weeks and then come back for laser treatment. Derik typed out his speech for the thanksgiving ceremony in large type on his computer, but by the time of the gathering he could no longer read even the large letters. Yet he knew exactly what he wanted to say.

Our friends Francois and Antoinette offered us the use of their tasting venue on the wine estate, Simonsig. My colleague Anette designed the invitations; Griet arranged for white tablecloths; Anette C brought two chandeliers with white candles and also placed one small white candle with a single arum lily on each table. Antoinette did a huge arrangement of arum lilies at the entrance; Theunis baked bread and brought wine for the communion; Deon, Bart and Hans saw to the barbecue; Marjanne made salads and our mothers provided the trifle.

And so, shortly before his birthday, on Sunday, 12 September, with the help of our friends and family, we were able to bring together approximately one hundred people to give thanks for the love we had so lavishly received and also for Derik's life and the almost twenty years we had spent together.

Stellenbosch
12 September 1999

Dear friends and family

Whenever I think of you, I see God's love, His truth and His light in your deeds. Your unconditional love towards us is proof that there is perfection in everything.

Therefore I want to thank each of you for your loving care.

Since Derik was diagnosed and particularly since he was hospitalised in November you have radiated a strength and a warmth that still enrich us daily. You make God's love visible. You enfold us in your warmth with your prayers and with your positive energy, by giving us rusks, fruit, wine, cards, flowers, plants, music, candles, many hugs, warm dinners and a gift voucher for aromatherapy. Thank you for togetherness around a table with you and your children, for mowing our lawn, taking care of our swimming pool, repairing lights, a car, doorbells and doors, making phone calls, leaving messages, running errands, lending your wonderful support at work, visiting Derik in hospital and at home, providing willing shoulders when I call, giving the right books at the right time, a hot water bottle between my sheets, a pill at my bedside, long conversations… and for simply always being there. You pray, believe, accept and discover with us. You were, and still are, with us.

Shortly after we heard that Derik could no longer be treated, a colleague from Botswana suggested that I read Psalm 23 again and again:

"Fear not, for I am with you … In your darkest hour, I will be your light. In your blackest moment, I will be your consolation. In your most difficult and trying time, I will be your strength. Therefore, have faith! For I am your shepherd; you shall not want. I will cause you to lie down in green pastures; I will lead you beside still waters.

I will restore your soul, and lead you in the paths of righteousness for My Name's sake.

And yea, though you walk through the valley of the Shadow of Death, you will fear **no** evil, for I am with you. My rod and My staff **will** comfort you. I am preparing a table before you in the presence of your enemies. I shall anoint your head with oil. Your cup will run over.

Surely, goodness and mercy will follow you all the days of your life, and you will dwell in My house – and in My heart – for ever."*

Derik's illness is the kind of experience that I feared with all my might earlier in my life. Now I know that there is nothing to fear. Not even death, for Love is greater than all fear.

The process through which we are going is indeed perfect. We can now appreciate the wonder of each day. Thank you, each and every one of you, for your part in that.

Marthie

We started our thanksgiving ceremony by playing the powerful musical arrangement of 1 Corinthians 13 from the film *Trois Couleurs: Bleu*. While we were sitting on one side, waiting for everyone to become quiet as the intensity of the music filled the room, Derik began to cry beside me. I held his hand and tried to control my own heartbeat. We both knew that we were there to give thanks, that this was the day on which we could pay homage to God and to our loved ones. Together, we wanted to confirm the greatest message of faith, hope and love. Therefore we did not want our own emotions to attract any attention.

When the music ended, I read the same passage from the Bible. It was extremely difficult for me to stand up straight and to keep my voice even.

---

* Walsch, N. D. 1995. *Conversations with God, Book 2.* Hodder & Stoughton, pp. 153-154.

After my reading, Derik stood up and explained that faith, hope and love all had a temporal perspective. Faith, he said, is the historical perspective and is based on the knowledge and experience of who God is; hope offers a perspective of the future and is founded on trust in what God was able to do, while love is the present perspective and is based on God's will. And of these three perspectives, the present is the most important:

"And now:
faith, hope and love remain,
these three.
And the greatest of these is
love!"
(1 Cor. 13:13)

He explained the relationship between love and God's will with reference to 1 Kings 19, which describes how Elijah hid under a bush, as well as the imperative to love one's neighbour as oneself and Christ's words on the cross.

After that, one of our godchildren, Anna-Marie, and her brother Peter, lit the large round candle that Sandra had given to us the previous Christmas. While the three wicks – representing faith, hope and love – burned, I read these words on Derik's behalf:

our friends

together, you are the authors of my life
of voyages of discovery in the universe
together we learn, ponder, wonder
and marvel at the immensity of the creation

the candle in my eyes is fading
but the experiences of yesterday and the day before still burn
   brightly in my memory

as we brave the rapids on the Orange River together*
we know that the Storms River also offers shelter at
    Mooibaai and Bloubaai†
together we light a candle in the Dom church in Utrecht ‡
its scent reminds us of togetherness, of philosophising
    together
we drink to spring with all its fragrances
a new season of growth that envelops us

on the waves of the air currents
we shared our passion for flying
and in the pain of the final kilometres
we knew that it was only the start of our next marathon

together we savour the blessings of Africa
enjoy a glass of red before the fire away from winter's wet
or simply succumb to crayfish and *perlemoen*
without wondering about yesterday or tomorrow

we swam, we dived as if we were still children
we walked, we ran as if the world belonged to us
at times, we paused our film
to experience raising your children

cleaning a pool, turning a screw
preparing a special meal for us
a telephone call, replacing a bulb
all make you a very special group of people
our friends

---

* Orange River = Gariep River.
† Beautiful Bay and Blue Bay - bays found along the Otter Trail along the Eastern Cape coast of South Africa.
‡ The Netherlands.

We closed by sharing communion and enjoying a delicious meal with our friends and family. The glowing energy of that evening remained with us for many days.

11

A Shift in Time

What is time?

Where does the past end, how long is the present and when does the future begin?

The hospital experience lay far behind us, and the three months since Derik had been discharged felt like a lifetime. What would the future hold? Despite his deteriorating eyesight, Derik continued to write on his computer. One day, I received an e-mail at work; it contained a piece he called "my darling wife".

It was the fifth verse especially that tugged at my heart:

> you coloured the shades of our lives
> your fine hands shaped the potter's clay directing our existence
> so that I could enter the fourth dimension
> where sound and music mingle with angel choirs
> without the cacophony of man-made mammon

Tears welled up in my eyes as I sat at my desk, unable to react. I wanted to respond, but my hands lay still, my keyboard untouched. Eventually, I did try to formulate a reply:

September 1999

I sit here, filled with emotion, my fingers numb
My heart yearns for you, my soul wants to touch you
Where are you, where is the light in your eyes
In which dimension do you exist?

I saw you between white sheets
in almost every one of the eight beds
in a single passage
with a body that boiled and glowed and shivered and shook

I saw the old world through your new eyes
Felt the grass, smelled the air
Tasted my body heat against your ribs
Renewed my inner being in your emotion

I see you now with hesitant feet but with a sure tread
You never look back, you forge ahead
I know that together we left an old life behind
To now enter, excitedly, our fourth dimension

But the worst still lay ahead. Derik could not decipher my reply on the computer screen and so he asked me to read it to him over the telephone. It took me a very long time to read the few lines to him. It was an extremely difficult and intensely emotional task. My words made it clear that I did not know what the future held and that I had started to sense that Derik was entering a new dimension. I also knew intuitively that I stood before a fourth dimension myself, although I had no idea what it entailed. Through my words, I thus recognised the actuality of a new reality. Writing it down was one thing, but reading the words to my husband was quite something else. Now I could no longer hide behind the safety of the written word, because speaking my thoughts out aloud made them concrete and direct.

Various occurrences made me aware of the shift in time. We still had regular contact with the nursing staff at the bone marrow transplant clinic. They would call every now and then to enquire after Derik. One day I spoke to Savy. As usual, I asked her how Wouter was doing after having finally received a successful transplant. "He died," she replied. It was a tremendous shock to me. Everything had been going so smoothly for him since he had been diagnosed correctly. It was only just before his transplant that his lungs had also started giving him trouble. Now he was dead.

We received more unexpected news – both items from Potchefstroom. A university acquaintance in his early forties had been killed in a car accident and my aunt had died after a short illness. This, along with the fact that Derik was still alive, made me realise that death does not always come at a logical, predictable moment. Unexpected things happen, while what we expect does not.

We also began to realise that time could not be captured in a single moment. When Derik was in the hospital, we could recall previous experiences just by thinking about them. The pace at which things happen also has nothing to do with time. For instance, in the space of a couple of months, we had advanced light years in the way in which we thought about life. On the one hand our thought patterns had developed far quicker than normal, but at the same time, our daily existence since Derik's discharge seemed to be happening in slow motion. At times, late at night, I became aware of Derik's warm, peaceful touch as he held me in our sleep. We always touched each other in bed, but these moments were like stills caught on a film screen. They made me look, feel and imbibe. Somewhere between sleeping and waking, I knew that I had to enjoy these experiences – it was as if our being together had never disappeared and would be there for ever. But at the same time I thought that I needed to etch these moments into my memory so that I could have them always – this melting together of our bodies, the safety of each other's arms. When I was properly awake again, the night-time feeling seemed strange to me – why did I experience Derik's touch so intensely and want to etch it into my memory?

Perhaps it was fitting, therefore, to start speaking of a new dimension rather than of the past, the present and the future. At this stage we were unable to describe the shift accurately. All that seemed clear was the change in our thoughts and in time. We did not know where everything would lead us. Derik regularly commented that he did not want to die and that he also did not feel like someone who was dying. When the owners of our regular coffee shop departed for the Netherlands temporarily, we bid each other farewell feeling sure that we would see each other again. They recommended that Derik drink chicken soup to retain his strength. We accepted their advice with gratitude, knowing that they were trying their best to be helpful.

Nonetheless, Derik started divesting himself of his possessions. He gave away his motor cycle, some of his tools and a pocket knife from World War II. When the Du Plooys came to visit from Windhoek, he gave Piet a magnum of wine that had been made especially for the 1995 Rugby World Cup.

The gardenia at our front door, which had been covered in gorgeous white flowers and green leaves year after year, started pining. The tree was filled with buds in expectation of spring, and did not lack food or water, yet it was not thriving. The branches with the buds drooped as if the plant was drying out. I tried everything to make it recover, but to no avail.

Since early September, shortly after he had stopped working, Derik had been suffering from intermittent bladder infections. The first time the infection occurred he thought he was dying. It happened on a Friday evening when we had planned a casual evening of hamburgers and videos. Although this sounds pretty ordinary, it was a special occasion for us as it had been more than a year since we had been able to do this. But it turned out differently. Derik experienced severe pain and discomfort. We did not know what the cause was, or where it would end, but we both instantly remembered his pain in the hospital. For the last time he made sure that his will was in order, that I knew where all our documents were kept and he sent a final e-mail to his secretary and to me. By the time the doctor arrived, he was doubled up in pain. We were extremely grateful for the help and relief Derik felt once the blockage had been removed from his urinary tract.

While the doctor was attending to Derik, our cat started running nervously around the room. I was helping the doctor and so I could not pay attention to her immediately. Only later did I notice that she had wet the floor – this for the first time in the five years since she joined us.

As always during a crisis, I tried to ensure that I did what was necessary without becoming emotional. I discovered how inured I had become the following afternoon when I watched a video we had rented, *Saving Private Ryan*, without batting an eyelid. We had avoided going to see it when it was on the film circuit because of the high level of violence. Under normal circumstances, I would not watch violent movies, but now I did not find any of the scenes too disturbing. On one level, I was staggered at the ability humans have to adapt to stressful situations and to survive. Although there are many examples of this throughout history, people are nonetheless amazed to discover when they are also capable of doing so. So too, Derik's pain and anxiety tightly gripped my own being, but it did not overwhelm me.

The bladder infection recurred more frequently, and Katerina wet the floor more often. I took her to a veterinarian, who diagnosed a bladder infection that had evidently been caused by stress.

Johann, our doctor, had to call on us more regularly at night. Why the infection and the accompanying pain occurred mostly at night, I have no idea. To make things easier, I gave Johann a key to the house so that he could let himself in whenever necessary. One night he was not available, so his colleague, Tienie, also a friend of ours, came over instead. Derik was in tremendous pain. When the injection did not help, she set up a morphine drip. Tienie and her family were on their way to their beach house in Betty's Bay for the weekend. As they were leaving, she and her husband hugged me tightly. I could tell that they did not think that they would see Derik again. But I knew this was not true.

The following day a gale raged around the house. As a friend who had done some urgent shopping for me was delivering the parcels at the front door, a door leading to the rest of the house banged shut with such force that a metre-long piece of plaster fell out of the door frame onto the floor. Later, when our friend Piet came to say good-bye to us (he was on his way to a book fair in Europe), I assured him that he would be back in time to see Derik again. I felt quite confident of this because on the Friday evening before our thanksgiving ceremony at Simonsig, Derik had also needed help with the bladder infection, and by the Sunday the doctor had been able to remove the catheter and Derik had felt much better.

On 16 September, a week after the thanksgiving service and a day after Derik's forty-third birthday, his mother returned to Pretoria for a family wedding. Once again, we were unable to attend this event as the viscosity of Derik's blood was so high that the change in air pressure would have endangered his life. It was a huge disappointment as we had all looked forward to being together for the wedding – especially

Derik, who saw it as a milestone he had wanted to reach. When we realised that we would be unable to go to the wedding, we both wept. Derik felt that he had started to lose his quality of life. He had very much wanted to propose the toast to Pieter and Nadine, as had been planned. In the end he did so by telephone.

The morning after the wedding, and a week after the thanksgiving service, we were alone at home for the first time in many weeks. We woke up in our blue and white bedroom, and shortly thereafter I started to cry inconsolably. I sat on the bed, on my knees, next to Derik and instinctively took his hand to press it against my chest. Like that, in my pyjamas, I wept as I had never wept before, not even when we had heard that Derik was ill or when the doctor had warned me that Derik was dying. My heart ached infinitely over our mutual loss. It was now my turn to weep because we could no longer do what we enjoyed together. Also, at last I could allow my own emotions to surface. They washed over me like a flood.

As long as we had had people with us, I had unconsciously accommodated them by not openly revealing my feelings. Derik and I had always only been able to let go of our inhibitions and feel at ease enough to show our deepest emotions in each other's company.

I did not cry for fear or over Derik's rising leukocyte count; there was nothing I was scared of, not even death itself. I wept over the loss of our life together and over the fact that Derik could not work on his book as he had planned because his eyesight was too bad. Weeks later, I realised that this was the beginning of the grieving process. I could, and had the privilege of mourning at my husband's side over our joint loss.

Derik did not cry with me. When I finally lifted my face, he looked at me with intense emotion – as if he was staring into my soul. But he did not cry with me. He told me that we could not continue like this, that his illness had to go one way or the other. He felt that his condition was intruding into my life. I tried to explain to him that I was nothing without him, that his mere presence fulfilled a deep desire within me. But we both realised that Derik was right – our situation could not continue like this. We had entered the final straight and we knew it. It was Sunday morning, 19 September – one month before 19 October 1999.

We got up, dressed and drove to Vergelegen* to have tea. It was an exhausting trip. It took a great effort for Derik to walk from the car to the tea garden, and we had to rest regularly. We called from our tea table in the garden to find out how the wedding had gone.

Pieter and Nadine were already on their way to the Cape for their honeymoon. This meant that we could go out to dinner with them one evening. Once more, the choice fell on De Ouwe Werf. In spite of the fact that Derik did not have the strength to finish his food, it was a wonderful evening and we enjoyed every moment of it. This was our very last outing together.

Our doctor tried to prepare me. He told me that people who suffer from leukaemia invariably die from kidney failure, severe bleeding or thrombosis. Derik, Johann and I agreed that we did not want to prolong the suffering unnecessarily. If it came to pass that he had to die, Derik wanted to do so with dignity. His only request was that he should not suffer pain.

When and how does one decide to stop treatment? Who makes that decision? A doctor is responsible for the body, and acts accordingly. But this does not take the whole person into account. A person also has an emotional side, a will, and above all, a soul. All these aspects have to be considered when one makes the decision to stop treatment or to continue

---

* One of the oldest wine estates in South Africa.

it. In this instance, three parties were involved – Derik, Johann and I. Each of us could potentially decide on a different cut-off point. I decided to take my lead from Derik – it was his life and he was the only one who could make a decision regarding his body.

One night, I dreamt that I was on the beach:

I am standing alone at the edge of the sea where sand and water meet. The beach is on an incline and waves wash over the rough bed of shells under my feet. The water ebbs and flows, ebbs and flows. And then I suddenly notice that as the water draws back over the brown bits of broken shell, they flip over to display their blue-purple backs. I realise that the rhythmic movement of the water helps me to see that the reverse sides of the shells are completely different to the front. They are the same shells, but their beauty – in my favourite colour – is revealed only once the water has washed over them.

This revelation brought me immense peace: change was inevitable, but it would be positive. Once more, I shared my intense excitement about the future with Derik.

Derik grew weaker and still suffered from the bladder infections at regular intervals. He frequently spent a day or more in bed with a morphine drip attached to him, but then he recovered again. He kept saying that he did not feel as if he was dying. He also started to get ear infections. The doctor let him choose whether he wanted to take an antibiotic or not. Derik decided in favour of the treatment and a within a few days he felt much better.

—— Original Message ——
From: Momberg Marthie
Sent: Wednesday, 29 September 1999 21:00 PM
To: Footman, Lydia
Subject: Derik

Dear Lydia

I am sorry I have not replied sooner. I was so tired on Wednesday that I stayed at home to rest. Today is Sunday, and I'm trying to catch up – I must tender for a project in Jo'burg on Wednesday. I think I'll work from home for the next while and only go to the office for meetings.

A lot has happened since we last spoke. The bottom line: We are both WELL, although we have discomfort.

Derik's leukocyte count is still rising and it was dreadfully high last Monday (256 instead of somewhere between 4 and 11, with 95% blast cells). During the past four weeks, he has constantly had infections and is now again receiving morphine. He has great difficulty hearing and seeing as a result of the enormous amount of fluid and pressure in his head. But he remains as loving as ever – just yesterday he still teased me. He also says that he does not want to die and that he has nothing to complain about. The same holds for me. We are both calm. In fact, just after we had heard about the high counts, I told my mother that I felt an immense happiness within me. I honestly have no fear. To me, this is wonderful.

I KNOW that Derik can still recover completely. I have already expressed my desire clearly – that we will be together happily, healthily and for a long time. I see us together in the future AND I LIVE ACCORDINGLY. This does not mean that I am not prepared to "let Derik go". If it is indeed his time now, there is a wonderful new dimension awaiting him. But that is for Derik to decide – and whatever he decides is good for me. That is why I still give thanks for every day and I remain excited about the future.

This was quite a lengthy answer to your question. I hope that you are well?
Love
MM

I had once more started working from home as much as possible, while my mother took care of the household. I did not have time to spend with friends, as I was dividing all my time between Derik and my work. The e-mail contact with friends and colleagues became a lifeline.

Friends like Sharon in Vancouver, Marietjie in Princeton, my colleague Anette and Derik's secretary, Myrtle, supported me daily in a very special way. They had the ability to run when I did, to walk when I did, and to stand still with me when necessary. They never tried to steer me in any direction and never forced an opinion on me. Without exception they were patient and full of understanding in their support.

— Original Message —
From: Van der Spuy Anette
Sent: Friday, 1 October 1999 1:06 PM
To: Momberg Marthie

By the way, I still haven't been able to track down the tape of *Jonathan Livingston Seagull*, but as soon as D is feeling better, I will make my debut as "reader-on-tape-without-equal". It's such a simple tale, but I really would like him to enjoy it again. Especially the part where Jonathan decides to return to the flock's outcasts and teach them to fly as they truly can.
Lots of love
A

To which I replied:

— Original Message —
From: Momberg Marthie
Sent: Friday, 1 October 1999 3:10 PM
To: Van der Spuy Anette

Dear Anette, thank you. We are indeed free. It is liberating to know that I (sometimes) succeed in giving Derik free rein. Fortunately, he takes them anyway. He's not taking any pills today – he wants to see where his body takes him. This is fine by me.
Enjoy work!
MM

A few weeks before, when Derik could still read, Anette had sent him a quote from *Jonathan Livingston Seagull** in an attempt to give expression to her thoughts and feelings towards him. With this, she reached right into to his soul:

> *If our friendship depends on things like space and time, we've destroyed our own brotherhood! But overcome space and all we have left is Here. Overcome time, and all we have left is Now. And in the middle of Here and Now, don't you think that we might see each other once or twice?*

Next to this, Anette had added: "Thank you for everything you have taught me thus far – we'll see each other again!"

A few days after he had read the passage and her words, Derik remarked: "You know, Anette really understands."

This text had taken him back to our student days when he had read the book and often listened to the music. Our friendly music dealer was able to track down the soundtrack, and within two weeks I was able to collect the CD and play the first two cuts to him on the last day he was able to listen to music.

---

*   Bach, R. 1984. *Jonathan Livingston Seagull*. New York: Walker.

Since he had decided that the disease was to take its course one way or another, he refused to take any more pills. Up till now he had taken handfuls of medicine at prescribed times during each day, but it had become increasingly difficult to do so. None of these could cure him, they merely kept his body afloat. By this time, he was permanently bedridden and his hearing was badly affected. The only way in which I could communicate with him was by putting my head right next to his and speaking very loudly and slowly.

As a result of the bleeding in his eyes, he could barely see anything. Whenever I brought him food, I had to switch on the bedside light – even during the day. Once he asked me whether our two engineering friends, Bart and Deon, could perhaps connect a light to the morphine drip stand at the bedside.

—— Original Message ——
From: Momberg Marthie
Sent: Friday, 1 October 1999 1:06 PM
To: Brand Myrtle

Hi there, dear Myrtle
I'm sitting at my desk at home – with the lovely yellow flowers you sent right beside me. We appreciate the support from you and everyone else at GS so deeply. You see to it that we never feel lonely. Thanks very much for the YELLOW (sunny, positive, expanding the mind) flowers and the gourmet chocolate. As always, you never stop making a very special contribution to both our lives. My mother also thinks you're the most wonderful person. Thanks, my friend.

Derik has been in tremendous pain for the past two days, but the doctor put him on morphine again and after an hour he's already more comfortable. He has a very, very strong will to live and today his hearing is better. It's just that the morphine makes him sleepy.

I, who stand beside him, have no fear, only a deep gratitude for the mercy of every day. And I'm so very excited about the future. I know it sounds strange. But it's a very strong and sustaining feeling. I am also not using any uppers or medication that could possibly make me feel this way!

If it is his time to enter a new dimension, then that is good. But I really don't think it is quite his time yet. I am NOT AT ALL worried about HOW Derik will get better – that I leave to God. I only know that we play a very important role by seeing him well in our imaginations. Our energy DOES make a difference. That's why I am so infinitely thankful that you are WITH us. Thank you for being you, and for the yellow flowers. Every time I tell D how positive I feel, he says "thank you" so beautifully. I will give him your message at lunchtime.

Know then that Derik is already better, but that because we are bound to an earthly conception of time, we are unable to see it yet. Just be patient.

Love

MM

Yes, it was true. Along with the visible evidence of Derik's physical decline, I still passionately hoped for his healing. I – and those who were going down this road with me – did not know what form this healing would take or when it would occur. The terms by which we normally determine time – months, days, weeks, hours – were units that could no longer measure our time. Every day was a lifetime, every instant significant. I knew day-by-day that Derik would not die on that day and that was my total reality.

Why then did I continue to hope? Perhaps I was more tuned in to Derik's soul than to his body. He still had a will to live and I refused to decide on his behalf that it was his time to die. As long as he wanted to remain on earth, I would continue to hope with him and I would devote my energy to him. In this way, I could continue to live every day.

Derik and I had both agreed long before that he would always let me know exactly how he felt. We often spoke about life and death, and I had told him repeatedly over the months that the decision to live or die was not in my hands, but that I always wanted to know what his goal, his intuition and his general feeling about this was so that I knew how to attune myself. If he therefore told me that he did not want to die, in spite of the obvious and drastic physical decline, then so be it. And if he continued to thank me for my hope, I knew that he needed it. Everything was as it should be.

He started hallucinating again, but this time it was probably because of the immense pressure of his high blood count. He had long conversations with friends and in his mind he was involved in meetings. During these periods of delusion, I was once more struck by his courtesy and his pure use of language. As was his nature, he was arranging collaborative agreements, praising team members for their good work and lending an ear to friends. He would for instance sit on the edge of the bed and say: "Yes... really... That is interesting... Yes... yes, I think you're making the right choice... yes, fine, Francois, thanks for the nice chat... I have to go now..."

One afternoon he called me urgently to where he was sitting on the edge of the bed. I had to come to drive the car, and I had to see to it that we got away from the vehicle that was chasing us. He insisted that I took over the steering-wheel because he was no longer in any condition to drive.

Just as before, he pointed his illusions out to me himself. Of course, I was well aware of them, but I did not see any point in telling him that. But I had underestimated my husband's self-consciousness. Invariably, he became aware of the fact that he had been hallucinating shortly after it was over. So he asked me to tell him whenever it happened. If necessary, I was to ask him whether he did not think he was confused. I did it time and again when I sat beside him in bed at night. Then he would become quiet for a moment and say, "Yes, you're probably right" and promptly lie down again.

In this way, we lived from day to day, unaware of twenty-four hours, but intensely aware of the infinities that passed in moments. Time and space were entwined. We were grateful, we hoped, we observed and we waited. The future was already in the past, the present surreal.

12

The Transition

I dream that Derik and I are on a long journey and that we need to stay overnight at various places. The dream starts as we are walking through an unending maze, searching for the address of the final overnight venue: we go down narrow, stuffy passages hewn out of white stone, without a window in sight. I am scared that we will get lost and realise that I will be unable to find my way back out of the network of passages. Our only solution is to continue moving forward and to find the place where we are supposed to spend the night.

Then suddenly it seems as if Derik is moving faster and with confidence. He takes my hand in his and tells me that he will find the place – I must just follow him. He seems to know where he is going. We turn left and right down side passages and then suddenly a sign with the street name is right in front of us. As the door opens, I see that the place is not yet ready because the cleaners are still busy. It is an uncomfortable realisation. They were expecting us, so why is everything not clean and tidy yet?

But then my focus shifts to the rest of the room. The entire unit has also been cut out of white stone – an exceptional work of art. I am struck by the wide-angle window that is set in the wall almost like a porthole. I quickly move forward to the window and realise that it is possible to see far and wide through it. I am amazed to see a huge stretch of rocks as well as the ocean in the distance. The surface on which we are standing is slightly below the level of the ocean. Excitedly I call Derik to show him the view from the window. Although the room is in an impenetrable maze of stone, it offers a vista of the world that is known to us. And yes, there are waves in the distance, but they are small ones that only fill the pool at our feet during high tide with crystal clear water. The clear, open view is completely unexpected, absolutely awesome. Then I also notice the huge, wide sliding glass doors to my left that enable us to go outside.

At this moment, I know once more that we will not be engulfed by the waves, that we are secure and that the water in which we are allowed to swim – whenever and for as long as we like – holds absolutely no danger. When we turn around, I see that the cleaners have almost finished the room and that they are nearly ready to receive us.

On a Saturday morning, during one of the doctor's regular visits, Derik asked Johann and me to sit next to him so that he could talk to us. He explained that it was time for him to die: his body was no longer of any use to him, thus he had decided to stop eating and not to take any more medicine, and he asked us please to help him with this. He also asked us to make sure that he did not suffer any pain. The morphine drip had to remain in place and he would continue to take intravenous fluids. Finally, he said that he did not want any more visitors and that we had to limit our conversations with him. We could ask him daily how he had slept and whether he had any pain, but other than that we had to leave all conversations and requests for something to eat or drink to him. This, he told me later, had not been his wish, but it had been his decision.

Outside, our gardener was pruning the bougainvillaea, and my mother was watering the roses that were on the verge of flowering. It was a lovely spring morning.

"You ran well," Johann said to Derik before he got up to leave the room.

I stayed with Derik. He cupped his right hand over my face. He could no longer see, but he wanted to read my face with his hand. He wanted to know how I felt, and whether I could accept what he had said. My face was dry and my voice, like my inner being, was calm. As the request had come from him, and since he had taken the freedom to make this decision, I could accept it. Up to that moment, I had hoped, but now that Derik had said that he was ready to enter a new phase, I acceded to his decision. He still was not a victim; he was not someone to whom things merely happened. He would die as he had lived – consciously and with commitment.

I remained with him for a while and then went to look for Johann. I found him in the kitchen. Johann was not just Derik's doctor, he was his friend. I put my arms around him and tried to absorb his sobs. To realise on a clinical level that a patient is dying is one matter; it is quite another to speak to one's friend about the end of the race.

"This was the first time I told him that his race was over," Johann wept.

During the morning, Bart popped in to find out how we were and to see whether there was anything he could do for us. Standing next to him in the kitchen I told him of Derik's decision. I wept, but it was not a helpless weeping of despair. An unknown calm had descended on me. The Lord must have held me very tightly during those moments and in the days that followed. I accepted Derik's decision completely.

The following day, I prepared a delicious meal – leg of mutton with garlic and vegetables – for my mother and me, and we drank almost a whole bottle of red wine with it. That we could do this within metres of the bed in which my dearest husband lay without food is still a wonder to me. Yet it is not something that I cannot comprehend. I knew exactly what motivated me. The best thing I could do for Derik at that time was not to give him food and care, but to give him the freedom to execute his decision without any pressure. By allowing him this freedom, I could **do** something concrete for him. By not holding him back or setting emotional demands, I could **help** him. It also freed me. Because he had informed me of his wishes, I could do what he wanted, and not what I considered to be "right".

I knew that Derik's physical deterioration had become unbearable to some people. One person thought that it would have been better to move him to the hospital; another felt that his illness simply had to come to an end. It had been nearly four months since he had left the hospital. He had not died within the expected time. Already for some time his blood count had been so high that this alone could have resulted in his death, and yet he did not die. Derik lived when he still wanted to, and now he was ready to die, but at the time and place that suited him.

Our home was a haven to him and I gave him my word that I would make sure that he was not taken to the hospital again. I trusted the process we were involved in and I knew that the right things would happen at the right time. My role was still that of supporter, and humanly speaking, only Derik could make a decision about his life. During all his fevers, hallucinations and pain, he had always known who he was and he did not want me to allow anyone to take this freedom away from him.

A few days later Derik intimated that I was not "strong" enough to help him see his decision through. On one level I could understand why he felt that way, because he knew how much I loved him and how badly I wanted us to remain together for a long time to come. On another level it distressed me very much that he did not know that I also loved him so much that I would allow him to enter a new dimension. Of course, it was not my wish that he should die, but I could accept it as part of the Greater Plan. I also accepted that whatever happened would be to both Derik's and my benefit. Because we had been unable to converse properly for the past two weeks, my husband was perhaps not fully aware of the growth I had experienced within myself and he was concerned that I was not ready to take leave of him. Therefore I broke our "rules" and asked if I could discuss this matter with him. It was extremely important to me that he knew that he was free to do whatever he wanted and that I would not hold him back. Derik listened to me and then genuinely apologised for underestimating me. It meant a great deal to me to know that he finally understood.

As often as possible, I lay with my body right up against Derik's. For as long as I had known him, this was one of the nicest things I could do for him. But being a fidget by nature, I invariably started wriggling and squirming long before he wanted to let me go. Now, I could lie against him for hours with my head on his shoulder, my nose against his neck, my arm across his chest and my knee over his legs. My touch calmed him and in some way gave him inner strength. A few weeks before, Derik had actually mentioned that if there was one thing that could cure him it would be this touch of mine. But I had to stop lying so close to him because huge blue marks started appearing on his body and I was afraid that my touch would aggravate the internal bleeding. Nevertheless, I always made sure that I touched him, even if it was only my hand on his arm at night or my fingertips resting on his shoulder blade.

I was in a permanent state of awareness, even when I was asleep, always conscious of Derik's every move as well as of the rhythmic sucking tick of the morphine meter. At night, he still held conversations aloud. Sometimes, he asked for a cold drink. Whenever he wanted to sit, I had to support him by putting my arm around his middle. Towards the end of the first week, he started asking for cold drink or juice more regularly and even had some of it. Late on the following Friday afternoon (six days after he had informed Johann and me of his decision to die), he suggested that we have fruit salad for dinner. I was extremely excited. Had Derik changed his mind? I rushed to the nearby fruit shop. The first strawberries and peaches of the season were on the shelves. Then I remembered how much he had wanted peaches at the beginning of the year and also my promise that he could have some in the new season.

That night Derik sat up and ate most of his bowl of fruit salad with gusto. It was his last meal. The next morning, he again told Johann and me that he wanted to die and asked us to help him by ensuring that he did not suffer any pain and by only responding to his requests.

He slept quite a lot by day, but occasionally he wanted to talk when I dropped in on him. When I asked him if he was happy, he replied that he was not really happy, but that he was not unhappy either. He repeatedly told me that we would be together again some day. One day, he – who could no longer see nor walk – told me how beautiful the house looked with all the flowers in it. I confirmed this, for there had been red and yellow poppies on the coffee table in the lounge for weeks. Every time the flowers wilted, someone gave us another bunch. Antoinette had also brought us a huge bunch of flowers from her garden on the farm that very morning, and I had put some spring flowers from our own garden in the dining room. I told Derik how beautiful the garden was – the wisteria, the freesias, daffodils, anemones and jasmine were all flowering and the roses were about to unfold their buds.

"I will pick you a rose," I said to him in an uneven voice, upon which he squeezed my hand in such a way that I knew he understood, for the roses were not blooming yet.

On another day, I asked him whether he was scared.

"I have no reason to be scared," he replied and then asked me whether I was scared.

I repeated his words: "No, I also have no reason to be scared."

We were calm and peaceful.

The only thing that disturbed the peace was the constant pain in his bladder when the blood clots blocked his urinary tract. By this time, Johann had taught me how to deal with this problem. Every couple of hours, I would wash out his bladder with an enormous needle filled with distilled water to prevent possible blockages. I was also familiar with the electronic device that regulated the number of drops of morphine, and I could turn it up or down according to Derik's needs. (The administering of the morphine was always done in strict accordance with the doctor's specifications.)

—— Original Message ——
From: Momberg Marthie
Sent: Thursday, 14 October 1999 1:06 PM
To: Colleagues and friends
Subject: RE: Derik

Dear friends and colleagues

It has been a while since I last spoke to you, and I want to bring you up to date on matters.

For the past two weeks, Derik has received medication for the pain – it is fortunate that something can be done about this. His leukocyte count is so high that no one can believe that he is still alive.

The most important thing I have to share with you is that neither Derik nor I are experiencing any fear. We are both filled with peace and gratitude. We feel safe and we trust the process that we are going through. We are incredibly grateful for the growth we have been able to experience in the past few months – and also for the role that each and every one of you has played through your prayers and messages.

I am currently working from home and I'm indeed able to focus on my work.

It is wonderful to be experiencing this wonderful weather – our roses started blooming today. Just as the plants rest during winter and gather food, we also get the opportunity to rest, to contemplate and to open ourselves up to new influences. Every winter is followed by a spring with new flowers.

Enjoy the beautiful day!

MM

It was a great blessing that Derik could enter his new dimension from home. I call it a dimension, for "death" suggests too much of a "final ending". I could also say that he made a "transition". Actually, that is precisely how I experienced it. I do not know whether he was aware of the fact that I was holding him. He could no longer hear with comfort, so I did not talk to him.

The previous night, Sunday night, Derik spoke almost constantly.

Among other things, he thanked me: "Thank you very much, my love, it was very, very nice, thank you."

Perhaps he was referring to the bowl of fruit salad. His day and night rhythms had been switched around for a while. Monday, 18 October, was the first day on which he did not sleep during the day, but lay there with his eyes wide open, motionless and quiet, except to tell me that his lungs hurt a lot. I adjusted the morphine. Something told me to stay with my husband all day. So I stayed close to him for most of the day – he was very aware of this. Derik was breathing audibly and with difficulty – a deep breath in, a pause and then out; deep in again, pause, out.

In between, I desperately tried to finish some urgent business for work. In the late afternoon, I wanted to go to my aqua aerobics class, but changed my mind at the last minute – again, it was as if something was telling me what to do.

I massaged the inside of his left hand gently. This had always relaxed him and his expression told me that he appreciated it. When I got into bed just after ten that night, I thought to myself that we would probably have a peaceful night because he had been awake all day. I was tired and instantly fell into a deep sleep.

But at one o'clock in the morning, Derik sat up forcefully, looking bewildered, and swung his whole body around to the foot of the bed. I had to stop him from pulling the morphine stand onto himself. And then he called out with great conviction and in a loud voice, "I ám dead! I ám dead!" He repeated it about ten times, emphasising the word "am" and shaking his hands up and down convulsively with his palms pointing upward and his fingers stretched out wide. As I sat beside him and gave him a sip of cold drink, I knew that he was making the transition (that is how I thought of it at that moment). Then he fell across the bed despondently, or perhaps desperately, and clamped his fingers around the sheets. To ensure he could not feel the pain, I set the morphine higher. At the time, it felt wrong to ask any questions or try to communicate verbally in any way. It was no longer important.

Derik's calls woke my mother up, and she came down from her room upstairs to the lounge. I went and set her at ease by telling her that I had turned up the morphine and that it would help to calm Derik.

I then went and lay behind him and stretched my arms out to both sides so that I could touch him from head to toe. We lay like that until I thought he had calmed down somewhat. Then I moved around and curled up in front of him as there was not much space. Still, I was able to put my right forearm, wrist and hand on his. My arm was warm against his cool body. All the while, I wiped large drops of sweat off his face. I remember realising that I was not at all cold, which was strange, as it was a chilly night. And stormy. The wind had not been as violent for years in Stellenbosch. The corrugated iron roof rattled and trees scraped against the glass and metal of the windows. I noticed with amazement that, oddly, I had been unaware of the wind for long stretches of time.

At one stage, Katerina leaped onto the bed and stood right on top of Derik. For the past week or so we had not allowed her to be with him and she knew that she was not allowed to jump onto the bed with him, but I could not stop her now. She stood on him for a few seconds, then jumped off and walked out of the room. She ignored me completely.

After a while, Derik pulled his wrist out from under mine and put the palm of his hand against his own chest. The fingers of his other hand were bent against his left cheek. I felt that he was distancing himself from everything outside and was withdrawing into his own self. Shortly afterwards, at half past three, I turned off the light because I realised that we could first rest a while. I knew distinctly and clearly that Derik was not going to die at that moment.

Almost immediately, I fell into a slumber. In my thoughts, there was a crystal clear image (it felt real at the time, and still does) of the two of us waking up together in a room in a house built of large stones:

It's morning, somewhere in the countryside, at a place that reminds one of a French or Italian landscape. Our bed is covered with pure white Egyptian linen and a down duvet. We wake up and our insides are aflame, just like the warm sun that is shining into our room. We turn to each other and then look outside. Through the open doors and shutters of our room, we look out onto a wide slate veranda with a bed of purple lavender around the edge and two dogs in front of our door. We are forever one, always together, in a golden white glow of light.

That is how I fell asleep.

The first sign of change I became aware of was when Derik suddenly started breathing loudly. Every time he breathed out, he used his voice. The previous day he had struggled to breathe in, and now it was as if he was blowing his breath out with all his might. At the same time, the morphine pump started emitting warning signals. I immediately jumped up to replace the morphine. But according to the meter on the drip, there was still some morphine left in the container. I thought it was very odd that the warning signal had gone off too early. I had replaced dozens of bags of morphine in the preceding weeks, and nothing like this had ever happened. Then I noticed that the fluid had welled up in the plastic pipes leading to his wrist. I gathered that his blood pressure had to be extremely low. Only later did I realise that Derik, and the Lord, had seen to it that the beeping of the pump had woken me up that very moment.

Derik knew how important it was for me to be involved at all times, to share, to travel the road with him. This was not only true for his illness, but for everything we had ever done. We always knew exactly what the other was thinking, and where we stood with one another. I will for ever be grateful to him for making sure that I was wide awake just before five on that Tuesday morning.

After I had replaced the morphine drip, I immediately lay down with him again. I held him, and at that moment I knew that he was breathing out his last breath. It was so wonderful, such a great moment and yet so simple. I touched his cheek and asked affirmatively: "Darling?" I wanted to say to him: "You have finally achieved it." I was immensely proud of him. And also of myself. I looked up to the heavens and said aloud: "You see, I am strong enough for this." I was intensely aware of his liberation, his lightness of being. He was still there, but without the depressing, sick body.

I cannot recall the details of the next two hours in strict chronological order. I just know that I consciously decided not to wake my mother immediately or to call the family. I know that I touched his entire body and in that way took leave of it. It was good to do so as I had not been able to touch him for the last few days as it had caused so much discomfort. I could sense his body and remember what it was like before his illness. I sat quietly with him, meditated, prayed and talked to him. It was peaceful and comforting. At some stage, I also removed his wedding ring.

When my mother woke at seven and made herself some tea, I knew that it was time to get up and tell her that Derik was no longer part of this life. We had tea, called the doctor and only later did we call the rest of the family.

It was the morning of 19 October 1999. My mother and I took turns to sit beside Derik's lifeless body until they arrived at nine o'clock to fetch him, as Johann had arranged. When they wheeled his body out of the house through the lounge, I stood up to say goodbye to him once more. How good it was that we had been able to experience all this in our own home.

13

Wind, Sun and Finally Mistiness

Around eleven, Theunis, our minister, brought his comfort and peace to us, and shortly after that, Hans, Anneke, Bart and Marjanne came over. We were all quiet in our grief.

Outside, the night's storm raged on. I cannot remember the rest of the day, but I do know that Susan was there at lunchtime and that more friends arrived at our house at about four o'clock. They came to hold me and to affirm their compassion by simply being there. Heather came and sat on the floor by my legs. At one point, she and I went to our bedroom.

"I want to tell you something," she said.

She told me that the previous night at about ten, while she was meditating, she had had a clear premonition that Derik was going to die. She saw him moving in the direction of a bright white light, but how an authoritative being – perhaps God? – had told him to turn around first and go and say his farewells. The following morning, she had another premonition, and this time Derik had finally joined a group of people. According to her, he looked somewhat bewildered, but the other people were very happy to see him. Shortly after that she had received the telephone call informing her that Derik was no longer part of this earthly life.

People came and left our house quietly. At about eight that night, Heather and my mother made sure that I got to bed. I moved out of the guest room on the ground floor, where Derik and I had been staying for the past few weeks, back into our bedroom on the upper floor of the house.

Holding a card that Hanlie had designed especially for me, I fell asleep. On the front was a colour photo of a single stem of lavender against a backdrop of more plant stems. She did not know that in my final image in which Derik and I were united for ever, I had seen lavender. Her words therefore struck me deeply: "… I photographed this sprig of lavender a while back – like us, it's a loner, and yet part of something else. The lavender makes me think of you and your love of flowers. Know that we grow with you on the lavender bush and that we share in your root system that is planted in God's earth…"

On Derik's side of the bed, the first white rose of the season stood in a delicate glass vase. I had picked it for him earlier that morning. Katerina came to lick the tears off my face – just as she had on the evening when I heard that the blast cells were back in Derik's blood. The tremendous wind continued unabated throughout the night, and also the following day when the rest of the family arrived from Pretoria, Johannesburg and England.

There were practical arrangements to attend to. Just as with Derik's illness, our friends literally held my hand and did whatever they could to help. Anneke saw to it that someone delivered meals to our house every day; Hans and Heather sat with me on the sombre chairs at the undertaker's; Anette C picked the most gorgeous flowers in Susan's garden on the farm and arranged them in the church; Tokkie and the rest of our neighbourhood arranged refreshments after the service; Strydom and Hermien lent us some white orchids for the tables; Hanlie repeated the lavender theme in her design for the pamphlets we used in the church; Elna played the organ, and various friends brought lavender from their gardens to hand to everyone as they entered the church.

Thank You

My best friend, my darling husband, my sounding board, is gone. It is as if a mirror has broken. Whenever I put a candle in front of this mirror, the light always shone back much magnified. The image in the mirror resembled me, but actually it was just the opposite. But it is shattered.

In the pieces of broken mirror I now see many faces – those of our friends, our colleagues and our family. As in the months of Derik's illness, you now reflect your light at me from all angles. You continue to help me with practicalities like making food, cleaning the pool, answering the telephone and seeing to administrative tasks. But you also feed my soul with your love and care. Your flowers and messages fill our whole house. I cannot thank you enough. May the Lord bless each of you in abundance.
Marthie

On Tuesday and Wednesday the wind howled; on Thursday the sun shone brightly, and on Friday, the day on which we finally gave thanks for Derik's life, there was a welcome cool mistiness in the air.

Theunis led the service:

THANKSGIVING SERVICE
Derik Momberg
16 September 1956 – 19 October 1999
Music: Mozart's Concerto for
Clarinet and Orchestra in A major
Welcome
Prayer
Hymn
Opportunity for friends to share reminiscences about Derik

MEDITATION

George Bernard Shaw once said, "Those who do not know how to live, must make a merit of dying."

Sören Kierkegaard, the Danish philosopher, stated "Life is not a problem to be solved but a reality to be experienced."

... upon which Martin Esslin remarked: "The dignity of man lies in his ability to face reality in all its meaninglessness."

But for me, the most descriptive passage about life, also as Derik lived it, comes from Marion Howard: "Life is like a blanket [that is] too short. You pull it up and your toes rebel, you yank it down and shivers meander about your shoulder[s]; but cheerful folks manage to draw their knees up and pass a very comfortable night."*

Thus there are many tongue-in-cheek remarks, anecdotes and proverbs about life. But when the preacher in The Book of Ecclesiastes thinks about it, he experiences a great paradox – you live, but yet you are going to die...

He says in Chapter 1: Man is made with the desire to discover things, to investigate, to think things over and to gather knowledge, and yet the answers elude him. He says that what is crooked cannot become straight, and what is not here cannot be counted, that everything amounts to chasing after the wind.

Man collects possessions, but at his death, he leaves them to another who has not worked for them. This is not right, he writes. What good has it done man that he busied himself so much with the things of this world, all amounts to nothing.

Man has a sense of time... and yet, yet he cannot find the right time.

---

* Quotations from Peter, L. (comp.) 1977. *Quotations for our Time.* Magnum Books, Methuen Paperbacks Ltd, pp. 304-310.

It is not the fastest among us who wins the race, not the strongest who conquers the war, not the smartest ones who become rich and not those with knowledge with whom all goes well.

Everything, everything in life is a great mystery, a riddle. He writes: "Then I turned and reviewed all my handiwork, all my labour and toil, and I saw that everything was emptiness and chasing the wind, of no profit under the sun" (2:11). Yes, one can gather wisdom, can think that one gains great power with knowledge, that one can guide life and even manipulate, can gather possessions and become wealthy and be successful... and yet, and yet everything comes to naught. "I hated life," he writes in Chapter 2, verse 17.

He comes to the conclusion that that which man is, is already contained in the name "human". We know what he is: he is human... and as a human he is confronted with One who is stronger than he... One whose work he is unable to understand from beginning to end (Chapter 3). He writes in Chapter 11, verse 5: "You do not know how a pregnant woman comes to have a body and a living spirit in her womb; nor do you know how God, the maker of all things, works." He does everything.

Yes, He is the God who provides rain to both good and bad. And yet, is it not simply man's own doing that he is able to eat and drink and still enjoy what is good in spite of his labours? I have seen that it is a gift from the hand of God.

Is this not wonderful? Life is a riddle, a mystery, but we should see it as a gift from the hand of Him whom we cannot capture in words. He who is stronger than all of us, who is unpredictable, whose depths we cannot plumb. Yes, He is in heaven and on earth. Our lives are confined: there is a time to be born and a time to die, and our bodies will return to the earth from which they were taken.

And that is why the preacher reaches the insight that there is nothing better for mankind to do than to be happy and to enjoy the good things in life. It is a gift from God that we are able to eat and drink and enjoy life in the midst of our labours. So we should take this gift with both hands and nurture it. He writes in Chapter 9: "Go to it then, eat your food and enjoy it, and drink your wine with a cheerful heart; for already God has accepted what you have done... Always be dressed in white and never fail to anoint your head. Enjoy life with the woman you love all the days of your allotted span here under the sun, empty as they are, for that is your lot while you live and labour here under the sun... Whatever task lies to your hand, do it with all your might..." Yes, enjoy the life that God has given you on this earth.

Be glad about this godly gift and go and be! Go and live despite the riddle and the paradox. "Cheerful folks manage to draw their knees up and pass a very comfortable night."

On Sunday, 12 September, we celebrated with Derik and Marthie. Derik shared a message from 1 Corinthians 13 with us and we were able to break bread together and drink wine and share our frailty with one another.

Derik said: In Corinth the people competed with one another. There was division, dissension and jealousy, but thank you to you, our friends... that we have faith, hope and love to share with one another. Faith, love and hope, he said all have a temporal perspective:

- Faith (the historical perspective) is based on the knowledge and experience of who God is. He is Yahweh: I am who I am, the God of action. He is also the God of salvation who can say even to the sinner, "I assure you: today you will be in Paradise with me" (Luke 23:43).
- Hope (the future perspective) is about trust in God's abilities – the God who was prepared to come and give us a new life in a broken world.

- Love (the present perspective) is based on the will of God … not in being self-absorbed, but in losing yourself in others. It is like a burning candle that, in burning, also gives light to others. Thank you for your love, Derik said.

    … and now: faith, hope and love remain, these three: and the greatest of these is love!

Music: Song for the unification of Europe
from Trois Couleurs: Bleu
(a musical arrangement of 1 Cor. 13)
Lighting of candle: Marthie
Prayer: Christo Greyling
Benedictions
Music: "Be" from Jonathan Livingston Seagull

Before we emerged into the welcome mist that followed the storm and the previous day's sunshine, Theunis read the Irish benediction that Derik had included in his final e-mail to his colleagues:

May the road rise to meet you
May the wind always be at your back
May the sun shine warm upon your face
And the rain fall soft on your fields
And until we meet again,
May God hold you in the palm of His hands.

It felt to me as if Derik was present in the church with us, as if he had watched over everything and then said to me: "It is good."

I was not the only one who had experienced his presence in the church.

When I opened the door of our home on my return from the thanksgiving service, Jan Garbarek and the Hilliard Ensemble's "Officium" was playing softly in the house. This was strange as the house had been locked and no one had been inside while we were at the church. Our friend Hans had given the CD to Derik on his birthday a month before. I thought that perhaps one of my brothers had turned the CD player on, but this was not so. I asked around among those who were in the house, as I wanted to thank the person for providing the perfect music at the right moment, but no one knew who had been responsible. Then I realised that it must have been Hans himself who had taken the new CD from its case and put it on to play. After all, he also had a key to the house. But upon enquiry, it turned out that he had not done it. I still do not know who turned on the music.

A full three months after Derik's death, the house still looked beautiful, filled with flowers that came from people all over the world.

14

The Thoroughfare

I miss my soul mate with my entire being – the gentleness in his eyes; the rich sound of his voice; the warmth of his touch; his understanding and acceptance of who I am; the comfortable togetherness in our house and our garden; the way in which we shared and honed dreams, thoughts and ideas; all the pleasure and fun we had, his particular approach to life. There is no way around, over or under pain, one has to go through it.

Gliding through the pain with apparent ease, or following a detour might make everyone around feel better and one can even momentarily convince oneself that it can be sidestepped. It is for instance possible to hide the hurt from time to time by occupying oneself with the everyday, or by consciously or unconsciously succumbing to the pressures of society, pretending that one's life has been shaken only for a brief moment. But one only fools oneself and delays having to work through the grief.

Experiencing pain does not necessarily mean that one has not made peace with the cause. Heartache and peace can exist side by side with equal strength, but the separation from a loved one remains intensely traumatic, no matter how much peace and insight there may be.

I experienced my separation from Derik as a concrete, acute, physical feeling. For instance, one night shortly after his death, while I was speaking to a friend on the telephone, I began to cry bitterly. I had been telling her that I had been (incorrectly) informed that it would be very difficult for me to keep Derik's company car. I found it unbearable to think of having to part with the safe and comfortable car in which for months I had enjoyed listening to music on my way to and from the hospital. It was almost as if I had to take leave of another part of Derik. During the conversation, I was leaning against the pillows on the bed, when suddenly I "saw" a broad current of energy, or light, rise out of my body: or rather, it was torn from my midriff and moved off in the direction of the ceiling, away from me. A tremendously intense pain lifted my torso and left me weak and nauseous. I wondered how much this sensation had had to do with the real withdrawal of energy between Derik and me.

But there was more to my loss than that. Being truly alone for the first time in my adult life meant that my life had been affected to the core. It was difficult to establish a new, meaningful structure, to fit into a new pattern. After Derik's death, I tried to continue with my usual routine of work and personal activities. But I was like a warped wheel trying to turn on an established track. Within a very short time, I was down to the rim and realised that my worn wheel was on the verge of breaking. I was no longer the same person who could or wanted to fit into the same old patterns.

I discovered that the pain also manifested itself physically. When I entered the long-awaited year 2000 after a short Christmas holiday and fell into a quick pace to get my life back into step, I developed shooting pains in my skeleton, thus at the very core of my body's basic support structure. It was an old pain caused by a condition known as ankylosing spondylitis. Twice before when I had had acute and extended bouts of spondylitis they had coincided with my being separated from Derik for a long time – during his military service and while I was studying in Utrecht.

Just as before, the discomfort in my joints was so bad that I could not sleep at night, and this in turn caused other unpleasant side effects. Eventually I realised that this illness was a physical manifestation of my life's shattered, emotional base. Up to this point, I had been quite impressed with how I had managed to juggle my work along with seeing to the estate, the financial decisions, the maintenance of the house and my social programme. But in the process of being busy, I had suppressed my heart's need to grieve. It was only after I started listening to my body and addressing the issues on an emotional level that I began to find ways to manage my physical pain. There is no detour around pain.

I realised this: To be strong enough meant facing my reality squarely, no matter how intensely it hurt as I moved with my shifting emotions. This meant that sometimes I suffered immense anxiety during which my entire body froze in shock, so that at times I still felt nauseous and weak to my core. Yet I was also aware of the deep joy and excitement about life that still lay pent up inside me.

Not only did I have to come to terms with Derik's death and the run of his illness, I also had to build a new life. None of these are easy to do, but all are possible. I undertook to stay with our decision to find the positive in this situation; never to indulge in self-pity and not to become engulfed by whatever happened to me. Therefore I had to be aware of any danger signs within me in time, continue to ask for assistance and take conscious measures to stick to these resolutions.

Today I know that although I have lost my fear of death, there is still much to discover before I can also take on life fearlessly. Achieving this is clearly a new journey for me. That is why my hurt may not become a part of my identity. If I work **through** the pain, I trust that I will emerge on the other side of it. Each day I actively and consciously try to go through the process of accepting and adapting with my heart, my mind and my will, and I am immensely grateful for the help and love I receive from friends and people in various professions. Above all, I know that I have finally burst from my casing and that I have started on the wider experience of life, the more intense experience I had so desired.

As much as I miss my husband, that much I grant him his new life and I do not wish him back in his earthly existence. It is my responsibility to start a new, meaningful, happy life; there is no one else who can do this for me. I trust this process also.

15

A New Vision

When Derik was ill, I envied him for being able to write about it, as I also dearly wanted to capture my experiences on paper. But my head remained empty and I had no words. Derik advised me to be patient; he said that the words would come at the right time.

A month after his death, early one Sunday morning, as I threw the white cover over our bed, I knew how I had to start. I sat down and drafted the outline of the first chapter – the conclusion of the first ten years of our marriage and the start of a "new life" after my return from Utrecht.

From there the text took its own course, and I used every available hour to work on it. I did not deliberately weave the story around dates and events, but as the writing progressed, I felt the urge to check some of the facts.

About a week or two after I had started writing, I walked past the filing cabinet in the study when most inexplicably it came to me that I should read the letters I had written to Derik during my time in Utrecht. I pushed the thought aside as it was already late and, after all, it is not very exciting to read one's own letters. But the next morning, I woke up at a quarter to five with a feeling that I really **had** to read them. So I walked to the cabinet and took out the envelopes Derik had put away so neatly. As I expected, it was rather boring reading my own letters. Why I was doing it, or what I was looking for was not clear to me, only that something was driving me to do this.

And then it struck me. At that time I had been planning to return from the Netherlands to South Africa in time for Derik's birthday in September 1990, but in the end, I had delayed my return because I still needed time to grow within myself. As I paged through the letters, I came across the one that gave my new departure date as the evening of 18 October 1990, which meant that I arrived in Johannesburg the following day. The "new life" about which I had then written, I noticed, had started **exactly** nine years before Derik's death. With his death during the night of 18 October 1999, he also "departed" and entered his new dimension on 19 October 1999. Along with this, I remembered that on the night of 18 October 1999, Heather had had the premonition in which she saw that Derik first had to return to say farewell to me before his departure. Could these corresponding dates of "arrival" and "departure" and my serendipitous discovery of them all be mere coincidence?

Two weeks later, our friend Sandra suggested we go to dinner together. We had been friends for many years. She had been our first neighbour after our marriage, and at that time she and Derik had both been studying for their honours degrees in psychology. We had kept in touch throughout the years, and were delighted when she settled in Stellenbosch after her husband's death.

Sandra was the chairperson of the Hospice Association in the Western Cape, and because she had also lost her husband at an early age, I looked forward to discussing my experiences and feelings with her. At the time, I yearned for Derik and I desperately wanted to make contact with him. The morning before my dinner with Sandra, on impulse, I sent him an electronic message. (Fortunately, his e-mail identity had not been removed from the network yet.) My reasoning was that in this way I could send my message into the universe so that Derik could receive its energy and respond to it whenever it suited him.

Among other things, I wrote:

—— Original Message ——
From: Momberg Marthie
Sent: Wednesday, 10 November 1999 9:27 AM
To: Momberg Derik
Subject: CONTACT
Importance: High
Sensitivity: Confidential

… if it is possible, no, if you want to, can you please make contact with me in a way that will let me know that it is undoubtedly you? It is NOT because I can't "let go" of you. I just want to HEAR from your own mouth that you are happy. Here where I am living now, it is very difficult to understand how one can willingly take leave of a loved one. I'm also working on my own transition. I think you know that I am approaching it in a very positive way, that it even makes sense to me in a way…

Without understanding why, I was convinced that he would respond to the message. In fact, I was so sure that he would respond that I almost expected to receive an e-mail from him. But after a while I realised that it was actually slightly ridiculous to prescribe how he should contact me!

When Sandra arrived that evening, she gave me an envelope with a card and a photograph in it. I did not open it immediately, but on the way to the restaurant she told me about the photograph. It had been taken some years back at her birthday luncheon, and neither Derik nor I had been aware of it. Some time ago, when she was on her way to a conference in Zürich, she had deliberately put this, the only photograph she had of Derik, into her handbag just before leaving for the airport. That was shortly before his death, and although she did not know of Derik's decision to die, she wanted to take the photograph with her.

On her return from Zürich, her handbag with her ticket, purse, and all her personal belongings, including the photograph, had been stolen at the airport in Switzerland and she had had great difficulty getting back to South Africa. A few weeks later, however, she had been notified that the police had found her empty handbag and that it was being returned to her. And so the handbag ended up on the aeroplane on the evening of 18 October and arrived in Cape Town on the morning of 19 October 1999. When she opened the bag, she found her glasses and the photograph inside.

Thus, on the night Derik died, an image of him had returned to South Africa from abroad – so that I could hear Sandra's story and receive the photograph from her a day after I had asked him to contact me in an unequivocal way. Were Sandra's story and the photograph, delivered on the day after I had contacted Derik, his way of letting me know that he was "undeniably" present, albeit in a different form? Or did I have to write this off to mere coincidence as well?

This was not the only incident that made me feel that I still had contact with Derik. On the few occasions when I had consciously focused on him and asked him to come to me, I had always received a direct, concrete awareness that he had communicated with me within twenty-four hours. Although our contact occurred mostly at night (the only time when I was not frantically busy), I knew each time without doubt that it had not been a dream. I had had the same kind of experience after my father's death, and now, nearly eight years later, I still irrefutably know that he came to speak to me one night.

Sometimes, I also experienced Derik's presence without having asked for it. One Saturday afternoon, for instance, I distinctly felt the air move across my left cheek – it was as if he had stroked my cheek. His nearness brought a wonderful peace to me. It was extremely gratifying to know that Derik was now fully healed, happy and very energetic.

But when one is again caught up in the tangible, rushed reality, there is no visible proof of contact with the invisible world. Deep inside one knows that there is a difference between a dream and real contact, but sometimes, especially in the midst of the everyday whirl, one wonders about the validity of one's experiences.

About four months after Derik's death, having discussed an important proposal with my manager at work, instinctively I had wanted to phone Derik to tell him how it had gone as I always had. He had always been very interested in my work, and right then it felt as if he also wanted to hear from me. So I sat down at my desk with my chin resting on my folded hands, as if I was praying, and asked him to come to me so that I could tell him how I was. Almost immediately I became aware of him leaning against my desk so that we were looking into each other's faces. He was wearing his favourite yellow shirt, and I knew exactly what he was saying and doing. But that was not enough for me.

"No," I said, as the tears silently streamed down my cheeks, my neck and my arms, "I have no proof that you are really here. How do I know that it is not my imagination? This time, you will please have to do something to convince me finally that my mind is not playing tricks on me." And with that, a tremendous calm came over me. I smiled secretly at my challenge to Derik. Was he not the one who had always been resourceful?

During the course of the afternoon and the following day I kept thinking about my request – still at peace. In the evening I went to my friend Rieksie, an aromatherapy and shiatsu massage specialist. Before my treatment, she and I spoke for a long time – also about the wonderful discovery that the complete reality does not consist only of the visible and tangible world.

After about an hour of massage, I was completely relaxed and empty of any thoughts. Then suddenly, I remembered that **she** had been the one who had initially discovered that Derik's spleen was enlarged. I was lying face down with my eyes closed, wondering with amazement about the connection between Rieksie and Derik. These thoughts welled up like bubbles that rush to the surface of water, only to disappear once they make contact with the atmosphere. They seemed to come from nowhere and to disappear into nothingness.

It was Rieksie who broke the silence about three minutes later. "Marthie," she said, "I have just had the most incredible experience."

"What?" I asked.

"At first I did not want to tell you, but I feel I have to. I saw Derik sitting right here with us." She pointed to the spot. "He looked at us calmly and seemed to be smiling, almost as if he wanted to say that it's good that we're together here tonight." I jerked upright. It made sense! Derik knew how much I trusted Rieksie, and he had come to me in a way that assured me that it was not my own thoughts that had conjured him up! The realisation shocked me so much that I started to cry inconsolably – for four whole days.

We believe in life after death, we know that energy cannot be destroyed, we even believe in the resurrection of the body, and yet, when something like this happens to us, we are loathe to believe it is true. Rieksie experienced a feeling of complete peace for herself, Derik and me. Although she had not known him socially and therefore did not have many memories of him, nevertheless she described him in great and typical detail. She has seen Derik in one of his characteristic poses, with his head bent to one side, fingers folded in against his cheek and index finger flat against his temple. This was also the position in which he had died. The man that Rieksie had seen was healthy and happy, and the clothes she described (I asked her about every detail) were in his favourite colours. Her image of a healthy, happy Derik corresponded with the images I had had of him after his death. I no longer doubted that it was possible to make contact with a loved one after his death.

Along with these experiences, and while I was writing our story, I realised at times that some events during the course of Derik's illness were more significant or intense than others, and I wanted to determine exactly when they occurred. I was stunned to note that every significant event was in one way or another related to the date of Derik's death – 19.10.1999. It is a date comprised entirely of ones and nines, numbers that denote "beginning" and "destruction" (1), and also "growth", "completion" and "transformation" (9) according to numerology principles. The number 19, and especially a number that consists entirely of ones and nines, such as 19.10.1999 can therefore symbolise the end of a phase, as well as the beginning of something new: the conclusion of old patterns, old goals, and at the same time, the start of new opportunities and a different way of doing things – a transition to a different time and way of being.

There was a build-up to the final date. Derik was discharged from the hospital after his third and final session of chemotherapy on 19 April, six months before his death. Ultimately, the side effects of this treatment contributed to his death, but his discharge had also given him the first real opportunity to rest outside the hospital since he was first admitted with AML. My credit card statement showed that our symbolic new beginning after the exhausting hospital phase, our breakfast at De Ouwe Werf, was on 19 June. And Derik's mother's departure for the family wedding made it easy to determine that my acute sense of loss had occurred on 19 September. It is also interesting to note that Rieksie was born on 18 October, although her birth date is registered as 19 October owing to an error by her grandmother. Finally, Derik passed away on 19 October 1999, exactly nine years after our "new life" had started, and after 19 years of married life.

There appeared to be a definite pattern to our lives. This realisation calmed me tremendously, since it seemed that everything was meant to be exactly like this and no other way. Throughout his illness we had "trusted the process" and had known that we were part of a larger, unseen whole. Now it seemed as if the unseen whole or pattern was symbolised by dates and numbers. I choose to believe that it is a carefully designed Plan.

I now know for certain that nothing happens by chance, and that there is a specific time for everything on earth. Derik did not die within two or three weeks, as had been predicted, but only after four months during which we had been able once more to do what we enjoyed together and could gather yet more memories. I also know that all of us, including Derik and me, are for ever part of one another in life and in death through the boundless love of God. Our main goal or final destination is neither life nor death, but Love and a consciousness of the Greater Plan. What is important is that we consciously open ourselves up to observing the unseen. If it had not been for Derik's illness and all the events that surrounded it, I would probably still be "looking," but not "seeing".

Yet I do lose this perspective occasionally, especially when I am very busy and do not allow enough time to be still and calm within myself. Then peace eludes me and I become entangled in a myriad questions that are based on my fears. But as soon as I give myself the time to slow down and listen to my inner voice, I know that not a hair will fall from my head, or any one else's, without the knowledge, care and omnipresence of God.

Because I believe that there is a continuous interaction between the individual and his environment, I asked myself what role I had played in Derik's illness and death. My question was answered when I watched the film, *Left Luggage*. It is the story of a young Orthodox Jewish boy who unexpectedly and tragically drowns in a duck pond. He had learned about this pond, which was situated in a beautiful park, from his young caregiver who had not only given him the confidence to speak again after years of unnatural silence, but had also lovingly introduced him to the many beautiful things outside the sombre apartment in which he spent most of his time. She had freed him partially from the rigid bonds of his parental home, but one could also argue that, in a way, his voyage of discovery led to his death. At the end, the young nurse asks herself what role she had played in his death.

Her elderly friend answers: "There are many accomplices in his death: the ducks because he was lured to them; the water because it enfolded him; the trees because they stood by. But you, you did what you could. You loved him."

Along with these insights, the Plan of which I had become aware, the realisation of my eternal link with Derik, as well as the continued love and assistance of the people who surround me, my acceptance strengthened and my adjustment began. Derik's illness and death freed me from the restrictions I had previously placed on myself. I now know for the first time that there is eternal Light, love, joy and peace in me. Derik completed the greatest marathon of his life and he qualified for another journey in a new dimension. Just as our life together on earth was temporary, I also know that our separation is temporary – we will be together again one day. Now, too, I can choose how to react to my present situation – I can continue to live in the past, or I can live now.

I dream that I have to find my way across a stream of water. It is essential that I cross the river because on a hill, on the other bank, is a huge house I must move into and it is filled with people who are waiting for me. But it is not easy to reach the other side because there is no real bridge and I have plenty of luggage with me. It is not the first time I have to cross this river, but it is the first time that I have to do it alone. I have to step onto a rickety wooden structure with inadequate railings that zigzags high over the water. I scrape together my courage and give the first step, then another, after which I realise that I cannot continue like this. I can clearly feel the wooden beam bending and giving way under the weight of my front foot. I cling desperately to the scanty railing and lift my head, only to see that the rest of the bridge has been demolished. The bent beam under my foot looks like a skeleton hanging in the air. There is no way it will get me to the other side, and I have to turn around to devise another plan. I shuffle back and eventually find myself on firm ground once more. And then, as I look at the river carefully, I notice that the water is actually not very deep, that it is flowing quietly and that there are sturdy, dark grey boulders with even surfaces sticking out of the water. All that I have to do is to walk across the stepping stones and I will get to the other side safely.

Epilogue

The Red Pashmina

It was April 2000, one month after I had completed this book. I was standing in the middle of a wooden walkway within metres of the water in the Amazon rainforest. It was sturdy and newly built and stood about a metre above the ground so that people walking between the water and the campsite's gathering place would not damage the vegetation.

On the previous afternoon a few members of our tour group (seven South Africans and eighteen Americans) had taken a boat trip to go and observe some monkeys in their natural habitat. It had been a wonderful outing that had included a short walk through the forest and a delightful swim in the river. I had particularly enjoyed the freedom of the water in which I could stretch my legs after the long flight from Cape Town via Buenos Aires and La Paz to the northern regions of South America.

These were the first uninhibited moments I had had in months, and it was totally liberating to swim away from the group and shed my costume just as Derik and I had always done. Perhaps that is why I became intensely aware of his presence right then and knew that he was sharing the joy of the moment with me. In the boat on the way back, I therefore sat slightly apart from the rest of the group, closed my eyes and focused on his presence. I was vaguely aware that the people around me were getting to know each other better and were exchanging personal details. It was only a day since we had met and our tour of Peru still lay ahead.

It was hot as we stood on the walkway. The clammy, oppressive tropical air clung to us. But the heat was of less importance. I listened in fascination as Constance (later, I would discover that she worked as a healer, trainer and clairvoyant from Martha's Vineyard in the USA) helped Anna and Mary to explore a potential connection between them. As I watched them, I realised that Constance had an unusual ability to observe the unseen.

After their "consultation" I turned to Constance and before I could stop myself asked: "Can you...?" but I could not complete the question. My emotions got the better of me and tears welled up in my eyes. Constance put her arms around my shoulders and drew me close.

"Oh yes," she replied, "Of course, I saw him next to you in the boat."

I pushed her away firmly. "What do you mean? Who did you see next to me in the boat?"

"I saw a man sitting next to you on our return from the island yesterday," she answered.

I had wanted to ask Constance if she could contact Derik for me, but the words had stuck in my throat and I had never completed the request. Yet she knew exactly what I wanted, even though I had not told her that I had been married or that my husband had died.

"But you already do this for yourself," she added, as it was obvious to her that I was in contact with Derik myself. Still she continued. "Oh, here he comes – this guy must be important because he comes with **four** angels."

Mary, Anna, Constance and I stood in the middle of the walkway in the middle of the day, rooted. And Constance started to relay Derik's messages to me bit by bit.

"He says you were very strong for him. You were his strength. He is very proud of you."

"Was it a difficult death?" she asked me.

I was still unable to speak, so I simply nodded.

"He says you did nothing but grieve over him."

Immediately preceding this trip I had taken some leave to stay at home solely to grieve over Derik. Again, nobody on this tour knew about this, and even very few people at home knew about it, since I had consciously wanted to seclude myself. I stood bent over, with my right palm on my chest and my forehead resting on Constance's shoulder. I think that my teeth might even have pressed into her shoulder as I cried.

Beside me, Anna and Mary held each other tightly, tears streaming from their eyes too. I had met Anna, my roommate, a week before, as the South African members of the tour group had first travelled through Bolivia. As Constance spoke, Anna recognised the Derik I had told her about. Later, she told me that she would never, never forget Constance's face and how she had mirrored Derik's emotions completely.

"He sometimes brushes your face," Constance said. I thought of how the air moved across my cheek and nodded again. This was yet another thing I had never told anybody.

The words rolled from Constance's mouth: Derik spoke to me about a number of matters, he answered questions that I had and Constance also commented on her observations of him. She grew curious and asked her own questions.

"What did you do for a living?" was one of the things she asked him.

What would Derik's reply be, I wondered. Did he want to be remembered as a psychologist, or as a business manager, or maybe as a minister?

His answer: "My life was my work."

To my question why he had had to die so young, Constance replied that he had pointed to his watch. "It was my time," she interpreted. "He says he was signed up to come to earth for only a short while and his time was up."

At one point she said with amusement: "This guy has a sense of humour. He wants you to buy a gift, but it's from him to you. He doesn't know if this is quite your cup of tea, but he wants you to have it anyway. He has always pushed you out of your comfort zone and now he wants to do it again. Of course, you will have to fork out the money, because he is not quite in a position to pay for it."

I laughed too. This was typical of Derik. She explained that he wanted me to buy something like a shawl that I could fold or drape around my shoulders. It had to be bright and it had to contain plenty of red, because, Derik explained, red is "the colour of life" and he wanted me to wrap myself in this colour for protection. According to him, I would know what to buy when I saw it.

Although Derik did not say it, I suspected that I had to buy this gift while I was in Peru. I knew that the shops and street stalls throughout the country were filled with the characteristic colourful red ponchos that everyone wore. Was this what he intended?

When we returned from the Amazon, Anna and I started combing the shops and stalls for the right poncho. But not one of them struck me. Without exception, the material was too coarse and thick and I was convinced that this was not what Derik had in mind. He had always had a penchant for soft, flowing textures.

One afternoon, our first in the famous ruins of the Inca city of Machu Picchu, I was sitting at the top of the steep stairway between the old city and the agricultural terraces. There I had a long conversation with Derik. It was the afternoon after Constance had explained and demonstrated to our tour group how we were all actually capable of communicating with angels, mentors and the deceased. Among other things, she mentioned that beings from the unseen realms can communicate with us through words, signs, so-called dreams, music and even smells. It is like starting an exercise routine – the more often one did it, the easier it became. Her workshop made me realise anew that I had indeed been having contact with Derik for some time.

Therefore, when I was sitting on the stairs at Machu Picchu and heard my own voice in my mind, I knew that it was really his words and thoughts. Nonetheless, there was an element of doubt in me and again I wanted confirmation of our contact. Just before I got up, I asked him to help me find his gift, as I really did not want to buy a coarse Peruvian poncho, but I was keen to comply with his wishes. At that point, some other members of the tour group joined me and we walked down to the tourist centre together, in the direction of the restaurant and buses.

During the three days we spent at the Inca city I heard nothing but traditional Peruvian music at the tourist centre. However, at precisely the moment that I walked through the ancient city's exit the sounds of Chris de Burgh's "Lady in red" filled the air. I started laughing out aloud. I finally knew that Derik would help me to find the right present and that his energy was indeed with me.

A few days later, during a tour group meeting, Sissy, the owner of an exclusive boutique in Cape Town, walked into the room, her shoulders wrapped in a bright red pashmina. She sat down beside me on one of the covered mattresses on the floor. She looked stunning and I complimented her, wishing that I could find something similar as a gift from Derik.

Sissy noticed that I was cold, and so she draped her pashmina around both of us. After a while, she took it off and folded the soft, thin material around my legs and arms so that only my face showed where I was curled up on the mattress. The warmth of the silk and mohair mix made me feel sheltered. Perhaps I would come across something like this when I got back to South Africa? When I asked her where she had bought it, she said that it was from her shop and that she had brought some with her (Peru was only one of her destinations). And yes, she still had one pashmina in this colour for sale. I thought my search had ended. However, we still looked at a few markets just to make sure that there was not something else I would rather have bought, but none of the ponchos I tried on offered me the same warmth and protection that Sissy's pashmina had.

On the last evening that we ate together as a tour group, I therefore proudly walked about in my bright red Nepalese pashmina. Constance sat opposite me, and while we were waiting for our food, she suddenly interrupted our discussion to look into the space behind me and said: "Oh, he is right here, right now and he wants you to know that he likes your red shawl."

She looked at me directly: "He is so proud of you. He loves you so much."

There were tears in her eyes. On 8 May 2000, in Cusco, Constance and I held each other's hands and together with the companions at our table drank a toast to Derik and also to the present and future loves and joys in all of our lives. A toast to the things we wished upon ourselves.

"I keep hearing the song 'Lady in red',* I keep on hearing it," Constance remarked in amazement.

"Yes," I responded with a smile and sang:

… I have never had such a feeling
such a feeling of complete and utter love
as I do tonight
Lady in red
is dancing with me
cheek to cheek…

---

* Song by Chris de Burg.

She did not know about my conversation with Derik on the stairs or about the song at the entrance to Machu Picchu.

When I had embarked on my journey to South America, I had deliberately chosen to immerse myself in a situation where I would either sink or swim. It was a sort of challenge I put to myself. I had turned down three tempting offers from friends to spend a holiday with them in Europe and decided instead to go on this particular tour of Bolivia and Peru after another friend had lent me a book about a similar trip.

I needed to find out whether I could survive without the wonderful support of my family and friends. I wanted to see whether there was enough energy and emotional strength in me to live fully once more. I also needed to clear up some issues regarding my future on my own, and without being able to account for it logically, I knew that the trip would have a defining influence on the rest of my life. I wanted finally to determine how I should continue my life after Derik's death. I had accepted that I would have to start a new life, but I had no idea how to go about it and no one could help me with that. Therefore I wanted to undertake something on my own, in a distant country. By distancing myself from my normal environment I wanted to attain a degree of objectivity, space in which to think and plan.

I never suspected how deeply I had thrown myself into this situation. During the flight over the Atlantic, and on the first night after my arrival in Buenos Aires, I realised that I was devastatingly alone and utterly tired. Would I have enough energy for this journey? Above all, I was sick with grief and I missed Derik immensely. If I could have, I would have taken the first flight back home. I was panic-stricken. Would the other tour members accept me without a husband? Was I strong enough on my own or was I now only half a person? Would I get along with the others? Would they get along with me? Was I still able to talk about things other than my recent experiences? Would I become the spare wheel? When, oh when would I laugh again?

I knew that I had to cross the river of my dreams, but I did not know how. Even if the water was shallow and there were sturdy rocks to support me, it felt as if I did not know which foot to lift first or how to manage all the baggage I had to take with me. I honestly did not know if I was even allowed to take any baggage with me. For some or other reason that remains unclear, I thought that I had to "leave Derik behind" before I could "make a new start". And I did not want to leave my life with Derik behind, but I did want a fresh start. How does one go about doing this?

Almost at the very end of the trip and after many experiences, I realised at a very specific moment that Derik would always be part of my life and that the fact that our love would never disappear did not prevent me from allowing new people to enter my earthly existence. It is thus never a choice **between** Derik and a new life, but a choice **for** Derik **and** a new life. Once I realised that, I wept deeply for the last time – tears of pure joy.

I am now on earth, and Derik is not. He can therefore no longer be my husband and friend in this existence. That is my reality.

When she saw my tears, Joyce (another companion from the USA) spontaneously produced her mouth organ.

"I'm told to play this for you," she said before striking up a most cheerful tune. She was unaware of the turning point I had reached in my life and had no reason to suspect that the tears had nothing to do with sadness. It was the umpteenth time that someone on our tour had conveyed a message from another dimension to me. It was as if Derik himself was playing the instrument as he so often had on hikes.

"There you have it at last!" I could hear him say. He was as pleased as I was about my insight.

Red is the colour of life. It is a colour of strength, vitality, joy, energy, passion and love. It is the colour of the here and now, the colour of survival.

I wrap my red pashmina, my gift from Derik, around my shoulders.

I will always be grateful to my companions on our trip through Peru – April to May 2000 – for their abundant love and assistance. With them I could finally weep my fill and start laughing again. Especially to Anna, Constance, Joyce, Megan, Mary, Sissy, Victoria, Beth, Jean, Margaret, Howard and Barbara – thank you. That which we shared will be with me always.